PRAISE FOR *OVERCOMI*

"Dr. Lee has managed the impossible: taking one of the most scientifically, clinically, and socially challenging conundrums of the twenty-first century and turning it into a great book that provides real down-to-earth help for all crystal methamphetamine users and their families."

—PETROS LEVOUNIS, MD, MA, Director, The Addiction Institute of New York; Chair, Addiction Treatment Committee, American Psychiatric Association; Co-Chair, Public Policy Committee, American Society of Addiction Medicine

"Finally! An unbiased, comprehensive, understandable book about crystal. Dr. Lee gives the facts and offers attainable solutions to the pandemic."

—KAT CORIC, BFA, artist, AIDS activist

"In *Overcoming Crystal Meth Addiction*, Steven Lee performs a great service by normalizing methamphetamine dependency. It turns out that this addiction, which has been sensationalized in the media, responds to the same mix of therapy, self-reflection, and twelve-step work as every other addiction. Lee's recipe spells hope for recovery."

—PATRICK MOORE, author of *Tweaked: A Crystal Meth Memoir* and "The Principles" on Yahoo! Health

"*Overcoming Crystal Meth Addiction* is a well written review of the history of this menacing epidemic and its devastating impact on victims and their families. In text easily understood by the consumer, Dr. Lee clearly explains the principles underpinning meth and addiction before transitioning to very helpful information about overcoming meth and staying clean. His five strategies for beating meth addiction are clearly outlined and a useful glossary of scientific and street terms as well as information on harm reduction and treatment resources are also included. Dr. Lee has invested substantial effort in writing this complete and understandable book that will appeal to a wide audience. The result is a valuable resource that bridges the gap between the consumer and the science of meth addiction."

—SCOTT LETENDRE, MD, Associate Professor of Medicine, HIV Neurobehavioral Research Center and Antiviral Research Center, University of California, San Diego

PRAISE FOR OVERCOMING CRYSTAL METH ADDICTION

"This is the most comprehensive book on crystal meth I've seen. It answers all of the commonly asked questions: what is crystal meth? how is it made? how long has it been around? how is it used? why is it so popular? what works in treatment? and how do people stay sober? For the person using crystal meth or contemplating using meth, it provides the most readable information regarding what it does to the body, the dangers of use and abuse, exercises for determining use and quitting, and resources for getting help. I highly recommend this book and plan on providing copies for all the clinical staff at all of our facilities at Alternatives, Inc."

—Joseph M. Amico, MDiv, CAS, LISAC, President, National Association of Lesbian and Gay Addiction Professionals (NALGAP); Vice President for Program Development and Community Educator, Alternatives Inc.

"Finally, a book that has a dual approach: stressing the danger of the drug and its addictive nature and engaging everyone—people in recovery, users, and mental health professionals—into a more contextual exploration of the complex factors that lead someone to fill up his or her life's 'holes' with crystal meth. Timely, informative and nonjudgmental, Dr. Lee's book offers an essential tool to examine the role of stress, depression, and unhappiness in one's decision to use crystal meth. It pays respectful attention to the culture of crystal use in the gay community and offers thoughts applicable to other communities affected by crystal. By describing 'the good, the bad, the glamorous, and the ugly' aspects of crystal meth use, Lee not only provides concrete strategies to stop using but also invites us to take a deeper look at the underlying causes of crystal meth addiction. This book is an invitation to a richer and fuller life, without addiction."

—Jean Malpas, MA, LMHC, LMFT, psychotherapist

STEVEN J. LEE, MD

OVERCOMING
CRYSTAL METH
ADDICTION

An Essential Guide
to Getting Clean

Marlowe & Company • New York

Overcoming Crystal Meth Addiction:
An Essential Guide to Getting Clean

Published by
Marlowe & Company
An Imprint of Avalon Publishing Group, Incorporated
245 West 17th Street • 11th Floor
New York, NY 10011-5300

AVALON

The information in this book is intended to help readers make informed decisions about
their health and the health of their loved ones. It is not intended to be a substitute
for treatment by or the advice and care of a professional health care provider. While
the author and publisher have endeavored to ensure that the information presented is
accurate and up to date, they are not responsible for adverse effects or consequences sustained by any person using this book.

Library of Congress Cataloging-in-Publication Data

Lee, Steven J.
Overcoming crystal meth addiction : an essential guide to getting clean from
CM addiction / Steven J. Lee ; preface by Marc Galanter.
p. cm.
Includes bibliographical references and index.
ISBN 1-56924-313-1 (pbk.)
1. Methamphetamine abuse--Prevention. 2. Drug abuse--Patients--Treatment. I. Title.
RC568.A45L44 2006
616.86'406--dc22
2006018149

ISBN-13: 978-1-56924-313-8

9 8 7 6 5 4 3 2 1

Designed by Pauline Neuwirth, Neuwirth & Associates, Inc.

Printed in the United States of America

For Ron, who taught me that imperfection is the most
beautiful thing about being human

CONTENTS

PREFACE

by Marc Galanter, MD

THE MAGNITUDE OF the alcohol and drug abuse problem in the United States is well documented. Eighteen percent of the population experiences a substance abuse disorder at some point in their lives, and the cost of addictive illness to the public has been calculated to be $246 billion annually in health care and lost work. Furthermore, at least 20 percent of patients in general medical facilities and many more in general psychiatric units have addiction problems, many of which go undiagnosed. Despite much progress in recent years, the addicted person still bears the burden of being stigmatized. When the secondary effects of addiction, such as cirrhosis, psychopathology, trauma, and infection are present, they may receive proper medical attention; patients' primary addictive problems, however, often go untreated.

Fortunately, important advances are being made in the addiction field. Basic research involving receptors, membrane chemistry, and genetic transmission has been elaborated. Public awareness has been aroused so that substance abusers seek help earlier, when treatment can be administered more effectively. New treatment concepts, both in medication and counseling, have made recovery a possibility for the majority of alcohol- and drug-abusing patients. Furthermore, the health community has been alerted to the need for early diagnosis and provision of comprehensive care. But the power of new substances to generate addictions cannot be underestimated.

Each generation seems to bring with it a new series of drug problems to be confronted, and, increasingly, each has its roots in earlier approaches to pharmacology and medical research. Cocaine was isolated from coca leaves in 1844, and its use as a local anesthetic was introduced by the surgeon William Halsted, who himself became addicted to the drug. Morphine was popularized during the Civil War to allay the pain of wounded soldiers. When heroin was synthesized in the late nineteenth century, it was thought to be a nonaddictive means of treating withdrawal from morphine. Amphetamines were first synthesized around the same time, and during World War II, their use was sanctioned by a number of governments, Japan in particular. Defense workers and civilians used amphetamines for their energizing qualities. In the 1950s and 1960s, the contents of inhalers containing benzedrine, a drug in the amphetamine family, were being injected intravenously. By 1970, the Controlled Substances Act led to the removal of these nonprescription inhalers from the market. By then, methamphetamine was already being abused.

Crystal methamphetamine has come to be a substitute for cocaine in many parts of the country and in certain population subgroups. Within the last decade, its abuse has inflicted great damage, particularly in the American heartland, where it has gained considerable popularity because of the ease with which it can be produced, and at a low price. It has become popular among some members of the gay community as well.

This book provides a valuable body of information on crystal meth, presented coherently and thoughtfully. It addresses the issue head-on by clearly explaining how methamphetamine affects the body, by enumerating the grave problems associated with its use, and by providing options for achieving recovery from dependence. It will be of considerable value to anyone who needs to be acquainted with these issues, or who wants an introduction to the interface between culture and pharmacology, and how drugs of abuse can come to produce major public health problems.

Marc Galanter, MD
Professor of Psychiatry
Director, Division of Alcoholism and Drug Abuse
New York University Medical Center

Marc Galanter, MD, is Professor of Psychiatry and Founding Director of the Division of Alcoholism and Drug Abuse at New York University (NYU) School of Medicine. He has served as president of several national organizations, including the American Society of Addiction Medicine and the American Academy of Addiction Psychiatry. As the Division Director of NYU's World Health Organization Collaborating Center and NYU's National Center for Medical Fellowships in Alcoholism and Drug Abuse, he has guided the teaching and training of addiction treatment at teaching hospitals and medical schools throughout the United States. He is the author of over 250 articles, chapters, and books dealing with addiction, addiction treatments, and spirituality.

INTRODUCTION

Justin **is a twenty-two-year-old** high school graduate living in rural Missouri. He works at a gas station part time but spends most of his days feeling bored, and frustrated that his life is going nowhere. The exciting scenes he watches on television are a far cry from life in his quiet farming community. There is not much to do where Justin lives. The closest town is an hour's drive away. He does not know who his father is, and he lives with his mother, who is unemployed and spends most of her time watching TV at home.

Justin started using crystal when his friend offered it to him one afternoon while they were sitting on the couch channel surfing on the TV. He felt amazing the first time he tried it because life suddenly seemed interesting, fresh, and vibrant. Worries about not getting anywhere in life or feeling bored disappeared, as even small things could catch his attention and seem fascinating. He stopped pitying himself and instead he felt powerful—he saw himself as a good-looking young man with the world at his feet, and his mind filled with possibilities. Sometimes he could become completely engrossed in a seemingly random activity. Once, he took apart his computer thinking he was going to fix a small problem he'd been having: Several hits from his crystal pipe and, twelve hours later, his computer lay in small piles of electronic pieces scattered around his bedroom. The place was in chaos: to an outsider, his room looked crazy, electronic parts strewn about in a mess that could never be put back together into a working machine. Yet, while Justin kept smoking crystal, it all made sense to him, and he was determined to get to the bottom of the computer problem.

Justin would hang out with his friends at home, and all of them would smoke or snort crystal together. Sometimes his mother would join them and get high. Usually she sat with them and talked, but sometimes she and Justin's friends started feeling extremely sexual. (Justin's mother has had sex with most of his friends by now, but Justin denies ever having sex with her.) One day, he found out his mother was pregnant, carrying the child of one his buddies.

Justin was upset at first, but he kept using crystal to try to make himself feel better, and he distracted himself with other things. Gradually, Justin started believing that people were following him. Even though he was in a small rural community where most people already knew each other well, he was sure that someone was following him. Although cars and trucks on the road were usually different, he was convinced it was the same person getting into different vehicles to throw off his suspicions. When he saw the people inside each vehicle were different, he decided there must be a team of people conspiring to follow him, maybe because of what he was finding in his computer. After he tacked up a sheet on his bedroom window to prevent people from seeing inside, he started to suspect that someone might have bugged his room with a tiny electronic device hidden in one of the little electronic pieces strewn about his bedroom. Eventually, Justin started to hear voices that confirmed his suspicions. He was right! But the voices were scaring him, telling him frightening things about what other people wanted to do to him. He became withdrawn and rarely left his home, too scared and paranoid to go to work. Eventually he lost his job and he stayed at home with his mother, collecting welfare and using it to support his crystal habit. He became a recluse, even within his own house. Before, Justin's life was centered on hanging out with his friends and complaining of boredom. Now his life revolves around using crystal, while he hides in his room, terrified.

Brian is a thirty-four-year-old gay white man who works as an attorney
and has a busy professional life. He is proud of the fact that he "works
hard and plays hard." After a difficult life as a closeted gay teenager growing up in a suburb of Chicago, he left his community to go to college and
law school in the Northeast and then moved to New York City, where he
discovered the gay party scene. Brian found gay discos and circuit parties liberating; they were places where he could be open about his sexual
orientation and bond with other gay men. After joining a gym and doing a
few cycles of anabolic steroids, he looked in the mirror and saw an attractive person, unlike the awkward and embarrassed teenager he used to
be, who had hidden his sexual orientation from his friends because the
homophobia in his school had made him feel so ashamed. In New York
City, he joined a circle of friends who went to discos and circuit parties,
where drugs such as Ecstasy, special K, cocaine, and crystal were the
norm. He considered himself a member of the "A list," a group of the most
attractive and successful gay men in New York City. Now, he thought, he
was someone that everyone else wanted to be. This felt so much better
than having to live a lie to avoid not being accepted by his peers. Now,
rather than be looked down on as a loser because he was gay, it was his
turn to feel better than others and to look down on them.

At first, Brian preferred Ecstasy when he went out, but occasionally
he would do a bump of crystal if someone had any, maybe two or three
times a year. Gradually his use increased to a couple of bumps every
month. About five years ago, when crystal was becoming more popular in
New York, he saw others doing it more often, and he started using more
himself, almost every weekend. He discovered that crystal made him feel
great and even more confident. He became horny when he used crystal,
and his main objective at discos was to hook up. Sex on crystal was amazing, and for the first time in his life, he didn't have any hang-ups about
being gay or fearing HIV. He just enjoyed the sheer pleasure of sex.

Brian began using the Internet to find hookups, and gradually he
stopped going out to the discos because he saved time just getting
crystal from his dealer and going online to find sex. An indulgence that
started out as one night of sexual pleasure quickly grew to staying up for
two to three days at a time. Instead of snorting bumps, which had actually become lines, he started smoking and even occasionally slamming

(injecting) crystal. He would crash and feel terrible on Mondays, eventually starting to call in sick. "Sick Mondays" became more frequent, and Brian's work performance suffered. He was given a warning by one of the law firm's partners. His prospects for becoming a partner of the firm were not looking good. He was not even sure if he would be able to keep his job.

Meanwhile, on the weekends, Brian continued his crystal-sex binges, sometimes using the Internet, sometimes going to sex clubs or sex parties hosted by his dealer. He'd often have sex without condoms. Sometimes he would start with a condom, but he would find it annoying, getting in the way of the wild frenzy of intense sex, and he would rip the condom off. When he was high and having sex, the only thing he wanted was more sex and more crystal, even if he wasn't able to get an erection. Sometimes Brian would wake up the next day with a very sore or slightly bloody anus from two days of continuous anal sex, or he would have painful abrasions on his penis. One day, Brian went to his regular medical check-up, and he was tested for everything. When his blood tests came back later that week, he found he was HIV-positive.

Ana **is a seventeen-year-old** Mexican-American teenager, growing up in a small suburban town outside San Diego. She was born in Southern California, the third of four children of parents who had emigrated from Mexico thirty years earlier. Her parents each worked two jobs, hoping that their children would get good educations and be able to have better lives. However, her mother and father were both busy working, and no longer being the baby of the family, Ana felt neglected by them, despite their best intentions. Ana was just a regular teenager who wanted to fit in. She went to school regularly and did fairly well in her classes.

Though there were many Mexican Americans in Southern California, there was a strong social pressure that "blond + thin = attractive." Social pressure was so strong that many Mexican-American high school students used to bleach their hair, even though the result looked unnatural. Ana was never interested in being blond, and she had always considered her thick black hair to be one of her best features. However, she became concerned about her tendency to put on weight and did everything she could to lose it. She found out from a classmate that if she snorted small amounts of crystal, she would lose all desire to eat. Also, on crystal, she felt so much better about herself that her weight almost didn't even matter. As an extra benefit, Ana found that crystal made her more alert in class, and she could get her work done much more easily. When she had a test or paper, she could easily stay up all night on crystal and pass the test the next day.

Meth felt like the perfect solution to Ana's concerns, and it was relatively cheap. Just doing occasional bumps, she would pay $40 for a little bag, which would last her a couple of months. However, the occasional small bump gradually turned into a daily habit because, on days that she did not use crystal, Ana became tired, depressed, and hungry. On those days, she also felt even worse about her appearance: looking in the mirror was painful. Over time Ana lost a significant amount of weight. Her plan worked too well—she was now not only thin but malnourished. Regardless, on the days Ana used crystal, she felt great and saw an attractive person in the mirror, and when people stared at her gaunt face and sickly body, she knew that they were really looking at her because she had become so attractive, and that they were jealous.

As Ana started to use more crystal, it became expensive to support her habit, and she began stealing. She didn't want to steal, but the trade-off was too expensive—looking and feeling terrible, and falling into depression. Ana was caught shoplifting and was arrested. The court mandated her to start a residential treatment program for drug addiction.

Justin, Brian, and Ana are case examples of three very different people struggling with distinct issues of crystal addiction. We will revisit them throughout the book to see how they coped (or were unable to cope) with the issues I discuss in the various chapters.

Crystal methamphetamine is an extremely powerful drug. It crosses social, cultural, and economic lines because it can cause such positive feelings in so many different ways. However, it can also have devastating effects on every aspect of a person's life. Crystal is an old drug that has been with us for almost a century. There have been several waves of epidemics of methamphetamine (meth) use around the globe, so addiction to it is nothing new. And now, worldwide, it is experiencing a new wave.

However, this current epidemic is worse than others because social circumstances in the world have changed: natural barriers that would have kept it more contained no longer exist, and other illnesses, such as HIV and hepatitis, make it more of a deadly, raging force.

In the information and technology era, ingredients to make methamphetamine are easily available on the Internet, so the drug is easier than ever to produce and to procure. As HIV continues to spread across the globe, a drug that causes intense sexual cravings and makes people ignore safer-sex practices continues to fuel the HIV epidemic, as well as the spread of other sexually transmitted diseases such as hepatitis B and C, which can all be deadly. The irregular and intermittent use of HIV medications by someone getting high frequently can breed strains of HIV that are resistant to the medications that are currently available, while researchers are spending billions of dollars trying to create new drugs to keep up with the changing virus. "Virus swapping" by people having unprotected sex and exchanging different strains of HIV make the situation even more complicated.

The Internet and the explosion of gay sex hookup sites in the late 1990s and early millennium made the possibility of finding sex while high on crystal as easy as ordering in dinner. In previous decades, people felt oversexed on methamphetamine; with the Internet, the possibility of sexual activity became almost limitless. The reinforcing effects of having sex readily available then fuels addictive use of methamphetamine even more.

The U.S. Department of Health and Human Services reported that in 2002, over 12 million people over the age of twelve reported having tried methamphetamin. Of those surveyed, almost 600,000 were current users. With a growth rate of about 300,000 new users per year, those numbers are much higher now.

The people who use crystal methamphetamine are found in all socioeconomic and ethnic groups:

- The working class in Hawaii, where this current epidemic is thought to have started, has been devastated by methamphetamine use: there, it is a drug that helps the plight of the weary, giving them energy to be able to hold the two or more jobs that many take on to survive the high cost of living in Hawaii.

- Unlike other illegal drugs, crystal has been reported to cross generational lines, with whole families using crystal together.
- In rural areas of the continental United States, one of the key ingredients for methamphetamine production, which is used as a fertilizer, is easily available in large quantities, and the open space makes it easy to build clandestine production labs. For this reason, the rural Southwest and Midwest have been particularly hard hit.
- Among teens, in 1999, 4.7 percent of American high school seniors reported using meth.
- In major metropolitan areas, many gay men use methamphetamine, and it has become the drug of choice in gay clubs and circuit parties. This has significantly affected the attempts to stop the spread of HIV in these communities. At one Los Angeles clinic in 2005, one out of three gay or bisexual men who tested positive for HIV admitted to using crystal. This percentage is three times greater than what had been found in the same clinic in 2001. Including all people who came to that clinic for testing, whether positive or negative for HIV, more than 10 percent admitted to using crystal—twice as many as had been reported in 2001.
- There have been reports of its use even in unexpected communities, such as among the Amish and Mormons, where strict moral prohibitions and cultural isolation would be expected to protect them from the spread of meth use.

Methamphetamine use is clearly growing, and its combination with other dangerous epidemics, such as HIV and hepatitis B and C, makes it even more frightening. It is a powerfully addictive drug.

As an addiction psychiatrist in New York City, I have witnessed methamphetamine spread across the city and devastate the community. Although recent efforts by the government and community service agencies have valiantly tried to combat this epidemic, there is much confusion and disagreement about how to address the problem. Some people want to dramatically portray the most extreme effects of the drug to shake people awake and cause some action. Others criticize this tactic as "demonizing" the drug and alienating users who see it as enjoyable, as the opposite of what is shown in frightening ad campaigns. Some people feel that harm reduction—allowing people to make their own decisions and teaching them how to use methamphetamine safely—is the best approach, whereas others feel that harm reduction just allows more people to reach the point of severe addiction, when it is too late to help them. The real answer lies somewhere in between, and this book is an attempt to find that midpoint.

I wrote this book for laypeople, to help them prevent crystal from taking over their lives, and for those who are addicted, to help them achieve sobriety. While treatment services are available—more are being developed and refined every day—the average crystal user either is not aware of them or does not want to use them.

It is difficult to know if you have a problem with crystal, and, even if you know that you do, it may be extremely difficult for you to ask for help. As you read this book, it will become clear that recovery from meth addiction involves reaching out to others and getting help from resources beyond this book. But if you are not yet at that stage, or if you don't believe you are an addict, you can also use this book to achieve a better understanding of why you may be using crystal and what it may be doing to you. If you are an addict, this book will show you the fundamental principles of overcoming methamphetamine addiction, no matter what treatment option you may choose to take.

This book is also intended for substance abuse specialists who want to refine their understanding of methamphetamine, the experiences of meth users, and specific treatment strategies for meth addicts.

My approach to overcoming crystal methamphetamine addiction involves five fundamental strategies:

1. *Learn as much about crystal as you can.* If you know what you are dealing with, then you will understand why it makes you feel and behave the way you do. Only then can you fully judge whether you are controlling your crystal use or vice versa. Also, if you know the physiological actions of crystal, you can strategize better how to fight back when it makes your brain crave more, even if rationally you want to use less.

2. *Take a close look at what role crystal plays in your life.* Is it something that you just use for fun, something that you control? Or has it become something that has taken control of you without your even realizing it?

3. *Learn the basic steps to stop using crystal.* If you are stuck in a pattern of using and you can't get out of it, this book offers approaches to stopping using, such as detoxing, something that many do not realize is a possible way to ease the difficulty and pain of ending a binge or a long cycle of crystal use.

4. *Learn how to stay clean.* What are the basic treatment options, including programs, therapies, and medications? What are some housekeeping tips for life that can lower your risk of falling back into using crystal? Even after countless experiences of the highs of crystal, you can still enjoy life without it—the book suggests strategies for relearning life, such as how to socialize without the drug, and how to enjoy sober sex.

5. *Make sure that you address major "holes" in your life that you may be trying to fill with crystal: depression, loneliness, weight control, boredom, sexual excitement, low self-esteem.* Using crystal superficially covers many gaps that need improvement, but if they are never addressed and actually filled in, then the urge to use crystal—your old reliable coping mechanism—will kick in and make you want to use again.

This book is divided into five major sections that follow these fundamental areas for overcoming meth addiction. Part 6 includes special topics that may be of interest to specific populations, such as people who have HIV, and loved ones of crystal addicts.

Overcoming Crystal Meth Addiction is not a blanket condemnation of crystal, and it is not an endorsement of crystal use. Like nuclear power, methamphetamine can cause powerful reactions, with some good effects, but it can also be extremely destructive. I attempt to provide a neutral description of what exists in the crystal-using world. To overcome crystal addiction, it is crucial to understand all sides to this drug—the good, the bad, the glamorous, and the ugly. Many people who have had good experiences using crystal understandably scoff at advertisements that demonize the drug and portray it as all bad. I take the approach that there are both good and bad aspects to crystal—people start using it regularly because something about it indeed feels good. Acknowledging the good experiences of meth is important because they exist, and a program that doesn't recognize this wouldn't hold much credibility for you. If you have to stop using it, there is a mourning process of saying good-bye to this intimate but often destructive relationship. In addition, understanding the ways crystal "helps" you is also crucial in identifying areas in your life that may need improvement.

Because of the extremely addictive nature of methamphetamine, I make it clear that the safest way to avoid problems with this drug is not to use it at all. However, many crystal users are not willing or ready to part with it. For those people, this book also serves as a guide to a better understanding of crystal, so you know what you put into your body; how to reduce your medical risks if you do use crystal; and how to monitor your use over time to assess if you are developing an addiction.

This book was written using current medical understandings of methamphetamine, the brain, and addiction behavior. In addition, I have drawn on conversations with and stories of hundreds of people struggling with crystal addiction, learning from their experiences of what crystal has meant to them—how it helped them with many things, but also how it has devastated many lives. They have also taught me what has been helpful to them and have shared with me their success stories, which I will try faithfully to pass on in this book. All names of cases mentioned throughout this book have been changed to protect people's anonymity. If you have recently tried or are even contemplating using methamphetamine, I hope that this compilation of broad experiences and suggestions will help you find your way to a life and lifestyle safe from the dangers of crystal addiction.

STRATEGIES FOR OVERCOMING CRYSTAL METHAMPHETAMINE

1. Learn as much about crystal as you can.
2. Take a close look at what role crystal plays in your life.
3. Learn the basic steps to stopping crystal.
4. Learn how to stay clean.
5. Address major "holes" in your life that you may be trying to fill with crystal.

HOW TO USE THIS BOOK

THIS BOOK IS written for a broad audience because so many different types of people use methamphetamine—straight or gay, young or old, male or female, blue-collar or professional. Many references or examples in this book refer to gay men because, while they form only a tenth of the total meth-using population, it is estimated that up to 30 percent of gay men have tried meth, and this is a community at extremely high risk (almost six times greater than the general U.S. population) for meth addiction. Nonetheless, I also want to clearly emphasize that *all people* are susceptible to the addictive potential of crystal. In addition, this book is meant for others who want to find out more about methamphetamine: a nonuser who is concerned about a loved one's crystal use, a therapist or drug counselor who is looking for a reference about methamphetamine, and even the curious reader who picked up this book purely for personal edification. For this reason, the chapters are written so that you can pick and choose whichever strikes you as most relevant or interesting. You do not need to read the chapters in any particular order, and I encourage you to read them in whatever order seems most comfortable and meaningful to you. However, if you realize that you are addicted, I strongly encourage you to read all the chapters, to get the most balanced and complete understanding of methamphetamine and how to overcome your addiction.

Methamphetamine has many street names, depending on the community where it is being used. These names include: crystal, meth, blue meth, ice, hot ice, super ice, glass, crank, Tina, Chrissy, chalk, working man's cocaine, chicken feed, and yellow barn. All names refer to the same drug: crystal methamphetamine. Some people distinguish "crystal" as a form of methamphetamine that is purer than the usual powder that people buy. However, most people do not make this distinction and use the term "crystal" for any form of methamphetamine. Because the names "crystal" and "meth" are so common, for the sake of convenience, these two terms will be used throughout this book.

Regarding the use of the word "addict," please refer to chapter 4 for a full discussion of what addiction is. The term "crystal addict" is used frequently in this book, and it is used without any judgment. There is no implication that the crystal addict is a bad person or has weak character. In fact, this book gives a strong message that addiction is a medical disease, similar to diabetes and hypertension, without blame or moral value. However, since the organ affected is the brain, the symptoms are manifested in feelings and behaviors, so it is difficult to see addiction as anything beyond personality. Like diabetes and hypertension, addiction requires treatment; otherwise it can be devastating and, ultimately, deadly.

Some may take offense at seeing themselves being referred to as "addicts." However, this term is intentionally used throughout the book in an attempt to destigmatize the term and make readers accustomed to it. There is nothing magical or mystical about addiction, and by reading it and saying it out loud, you take away some of the power that it has held by being a taboo word—unthinkable to say, and therefore unapproachable. Once you can approach the idea of being an addict, you have something to work with, and you can really begin to fight the addiction. If this book makes it a little easier for an addicted reader to admit that he or she is an addict, then this small offense to a few is worthwhile.

UNDERSTANDING CRYSTAL METHAMPHETAMINE:
Getting to Know Tina
Up Close and Personal

STRATEGY:
Learn as Much about Crystal as You Can

Objectives:
- Learn exactly what you are dealing with—know thy friend and thy enemy.
- Understand what crystal does in your body to know why you feel and act the way you do.
- Understand better what feelings are yours versus what are crystal's effects.
- Use your knowledge to strategize about how to manage crystal in your life.

BLUE METH, SUPER ICE, CRANK, TINA, CHICKEN FEED:
A Short History of Crystal Methamphetamine

METHAMPHETAMINE HAS BEEN around for a long time, familiar to different people under different names, including: **crystal**, **meth**, **blue meth**, **ice**, **hot ice**, **super ice**, **glass**, **crank**, **Tina**, **Chrissy**, **chalk**, **working man's cocaine**, **chicken feed**, and **yellow barn**. It's an old drug, related to **amphetamines**, though much stronger.

Amphetamines were first developed in 1887 in Germany as a diet aid, though initially they were not popularly used. By the 1920s, people started to use amphetamines to improve energy and to help with dieting and weight loss. They were later used by the U.S. military during World War II to help soldiers to combat fatigue during long hours of duty. However, their use was complicated by many side effects, including anxiety, agitation, aggression, inability to sleep when soldiers needed rest, and addiction. Later they were used as a panacea for such diverse purposes as weight reduction and the treatment of narcolepsy. Currently, amphetamines are still prescribed for attention-deficit and hyperactivity disorders, chronic fatigue, weight loss, and narcolepsy.

Methamphetamine, the more powerful cousin of amphetamine, was created in Japan in 1893, though as in amphetamine's early days, it long remained in experimental laboratories, far from public use. Like amphetamine, methamphetamine was also used by Japanese, American, and German military personnel to combat fatigue during World War II. Unfortunately, its problematic side effects were even worse than with amphetamines. After the war, military surplus supplies of methamphetamine reached the public market in Japan, causing an epidemic of methamphetamine abuse that was at least temporarily curbed by Japanese government legislation that limited the public supply.

Similarly, in the United States, after World War II there was a surplus of another amphetamine called **Benzedrine**, which was released to the general population. Benzedrine was used by truck drivers and others whose jobs required long hours. Amphetamine was similarly used during the Vietnam War to help soldiers stay awake. Upon their return to the United States, some soldiers continued using different forms of amphetamines, which served as an introduction to the drug culture of this country.

During the latter half of the twentieth century, U.S. pharmaceutical companies legally produced methamphetamine for domestic medical uses, as outlined above. However, because of the clearly abusive and addictive qualities of meth, after the passing of the Federal Controlled Substance Act in 1970, methamphetamine became tightly regulated and very difficult to obtain. This had a significant impact on production and usage of crystal. Production was mostly driven underground, into private garage or basement labs. Motorcycle gangs, such as the Hell's Angels, became major producers of methamphetamine, creating and serving a large market of illicit users. Often carried in the crankcases of motorcycle riders, it earned the nickname "crank."

Methamphetamine also gained quiet popularity among nonfringe members of society, including professionals, such as doctors, lawyers, and university students who needed to stay awake for long hours to work. It continued to be prescribed by doctors to treat obesity, though this use became tightly restricted, as it became clear that methamphetamine was an extremely harmful and addictive drug.

In the 1980s, there was a spike in meth use among the working class in Hawaii and California, with supplies coming from Mexico and Asia. Gradually, it spread eastward to the rural Midwest and Southeast, and eventually to urban areas on the east coast. Meth abuse became particularly heavy among people in rural communities, where its production is easier. The manufacturing process is messy, with strong, noxious smells, volatile reactions, and the potential for dangerous explosions. This is one reason that production flourished in rural areas rather than densely populated cities, where production would be dangerous and conspicuous to law enforcement. The ingredients to make methamphetamine are simple and easy to obtain, including substances such as over-the-counter decongestants and a common chemical used as a fertilizer, another reason for the drug's popularity in rural areas.

In rural areas, neither law enforcement nor the medical community were prepared to deal with such a proliferation of drug use. Some individuals in those areas have reported its easy availability as the reason they became addicted. Others have described using it as a way to combat boredom in small, isolated communities with "nothing much else to do."

Other affected communities included lower- and middle-class young women looking for quick and easy ways to lose weight. In a country where obesity continues to be a worsening problem, the social pressure to be thin has been ever-increasing. Crystal provided women with a cheap alternative to commercially branded diet programs and expensive gym memberships. Battling low self-esteem and poor body image, meth gave these people an artificially boosted sense of self-confidence and an ability to accept themselves, though this lasted only while they were taking the drug. Once they stopped, their mood and self-esteem would plummet into depression, their appetites would increase, and they found themselves no better off than before. Unfortunately, many found themselves on an endless merry-go-round of escalating meth use to avoid facing the body image issues that the drug so successfully hid. Even worse, the crash can cause depression connected to body image, which can make the self-esteem even lower than before using meth.

POPULATION FOCUS: CRYSTAL IN THE GAY COMMUNITY

CRYSTAL HAS BEEN receiving a large amount of media attention as a "gay drug" used by a subgroup of gay men in the United States. In absolute numbers, heterosexual meth users far exceed gay users, who make up an estimated 11 percent of all meth users in the United States. However, as far as the percentage of the community that has been affected, the gay male community has been particularly hard-hit. Estimates of the number of gay men in the U.S. who have ever used meth have been reported as high as 20 to 30 percent, in contrast to 5.3 percent of the general U.S. population. In addition, the association of crystal with unprotected sex binges and the prevalence of HIV make this drug a particular concern for this community.

Though the crystal epidemic started in largely heterosexual working-class communities, it gradually became a party drug for certain middle- to upper-middle-class gay men in urban communities, who used it to fuel their energy in all-night dance parties called **circuit parties**, in which some people would dance for twelve to eighteen hours. It has gradually become the drug of choice at these parties, which attract up to eighty thousand people, and which have become multiparty marathon events lasting for several days.

Before crystal, **Ecstasy** and **ketamine** had been the most popular drugs at circuit parties. Those drugs were appealing because they induced feelings of relaxation and social connection, both having significant meaning to a group of people that felt disconnected and rejected by a homophobic society. Gay men from all over the United States and from other countries converged on a particular city for a party, an occasion to feel connected and accepted. At these parties, they would celebrate their sexuality and embrace their sense of belonging, which was a powerful drawing force for tens of thousands of men. Favored drugs at these events enhanced the profound emotional experience of bonding and freedom; "breaking the rules" by using illegal drugs did not seem so bad, as gay men had already "broken the rules" of society simply by being born gay.

As circuit parties quickly became a lucrative industry, and the number of parties at each circuit event increased, the length of events increased from one-night dances to festivals lasting from three to seven days. Crystal gave partygoers the stamina to attend all the events and to enjoy extended holidays. Although drugs had always been a part of the circuit party scene, the draw these parties gradually shifted. Rather than being primarily a place where gay men could reclaim a sense of belonging, the appeal of circuit parties became more about the freedom of heavy drug use. Surveys showed that over 90 percent of circuit partygoers admitted to using drugs, with from one to seven different drugs used during a single day. The highly addictive nature of crystal increased the appeal of these parties even more, and for some, "the circuit" itself became an addictive phenomenon. Though people went to circuit parties with the notion that they were pursuing a sense of community, bonding, and better self-esteem, the positive feelings didn't last long after the parties ended and the drugs wore off. Many circuit parties that were actually fund-raisers for HIV organizations became events where heavy drug use and unsafe sexual behavior resulted, and this likely led to the transmission of HIV and other sexually transmitted diseases in many of the partygoers.

At the turn of the millennium, a significant change occurred in the way that gay men used crystal—more were smoking it. The circuit-party community, made up predominantly of middle- to upper-middle-class, well-educated Caucasian men, and the **rave** community, originally mostly Caucasian middle-class teens, used crystal primarily by snorting it. This was a relatively easy way to use crystal, and it was faster and gave a "better high" than swallowing it. Smoking crystal was initially looked down upon because it was reminiscent of the frightening crack epidemic of the 1980s that predominantly affected the urban poor. Gay circuit partiers, rave kids, and people in rural areas didn't identify themselves with the crack-using population. The stigma of doing something akin to smoking crack kept most people from smoking crystal, and snorting crystal let them pretend that they didn't have a drug problem: "We're not like those crackheads of the eighties. We just use crystal to have fun."

But as crystal addiction became stronger, people were willing to go to further lengths to get a better high. Smoking was the natural next step. "At least it's not shooting up," some people said. But unfortunately, smoking is almost as addictive as injecting. The amount of meth that is absorbed through the lungs is exponentially greater than what is absorbed through the nose, and drug delivery to the brain is that much stronger and faster. So smoking is a much more efficient way of using meth. And it is that much more addictive.

Not only does absorption of crystal differ from person to person, but the high feels different, as well. Some people don't feel that they have to stay awake all night, and they can go to sleep much sooner because the high doesn't last as long. But what comes along with a shorter high is a quicker withdrawal. When people started partying by smoking crystal with the intention of a quick partying session, many soon found that they simply were smoking more often, sometimes every ten or fifteen minutes, trying to maintain their high and to chase away the looming crash.

After breaking the barrier to smoking crystal, the remaining obstacles to heavier use were easy to overcome. Injecting crystal intravenously, or **slamming**, became more common. Crystal users looked for more ways to use the drug, and among some gay men, mixing crystal with a small amount of water and squirting the fluid into their rectums became a new method, called **booty bumping**. In particular, booty bumping constricts the blood vessels in the rectum, and there is less rectal pain during anal intercourse. This allowed booty bumpers to have even longer, harder sex as **bottoms** (partners receiving anal insertion) more easily, with the experience of having a "hungry hole" that enhanced or increased desire for sex even more. This also allowed for more damage during sex to the lining of the rectum, which increased the risk of catching sexually transmitted diseases.

Another major social change happening around the turn of the millennium was the explosion of Internet sex sites. In particular, gay-male sex sites made finding sex partners as easy as ordering food for delivery. Internet surfing, Internet shopping, and Internet sex (aka **cybersex**) were becoming their own addictive problems. Crystal meth, which intensifies both sex and other compulsions, in tandem with Internet sex sites became an unstoppable combination.

Internet sex sites developed their own culture and secret language, such as **PNP**, meaning "party and play," a code meaning that people were looking to have sex while using drugs, almost always with crystal.

This was also a time during which some gay men were becoming more complacent about using condoms. There may have been a decline in the fear of HIV because of the development of so many effective medications. The younger generation of gay men had grown up in the era of the "HIV cocktail": By this time there were already several medications to fight HIV, and many people started to think of HIV as a controllable chronic illness, like high blood pressure. Young gay men of this era never had the experience of watching partners and loved ones die from AIDS, so the specter of HIV was much less frightening. During the intensity of crystal sex, wearing condoms just did not seem that important.

A description given by a heterosexual man who used crystal illustrates the perspective of someone high on the dangers of HIV. This man had regular sex with female prostitutes, never used condoms, and he gave the following description of his experiences:

I was totally clear. I felt more clear than I ever felt without crystal. It's not like I was cloudy and fuzzy like with alcohol or heroin. It's not like I forgot. I still knew about HIV, and I knew all the information about how to keep safe and that I should use condoms, et cetera, et cetera. I've been in rehab and I've been lectured about HIV a million times. But if you think of a car rushing at ninety miles an hour, if you're on the street and that car passes right by you, it's scary as shit, and you want to run for cover. But being on crystal was like being in an airplane. The higher I felt, the more exhilarating it was, and the more determined I was to have sex. There wasn't anything else I wanted more at the time and I was like an unstoppable machine. Nothing was going to hurt me. And the higher I was flying in that airplane, the car traveling at ninety mph looked smaller and smaller, looking slower and less important. Really. Like when you look at little cars on the road from an airplane window and they just look like slow little ants. I still knew about HIV I guess, but it was like one of those little specks. In comparison to my need for sex, it just didn't matter as much. So why use a condom?

In fact, many people who use crystal don't use condoms while having sex. And this has had a direct impact on the spread of sexually transmitted diseases. In particular, rates of HIV and hepatitis transmission have increased, and various studies and health-care agencies estimate that about one-third of recent HIV infections have occurred during crystal use.

A Self-Destructive Binge BRIAN'S STORY

Finding out that he had HIV was devastating for Brian. Despite knowing that HIV is now a much more treatable condition than in the 1980s, Brian was terrified. However, instead of trying to take care of himself, he went on a self-destructive binge. He recalls thinking, "Well, if I'm fucked, I'm fucked, so what does it matter?" He went on an extended crystal-and-sex binge, using the Internet to invite men to his apartment over four days, having marathon sex without even stopping to eat. He does not recall how many people he had sex with, but he knows that he never used a condom. He recalls the sex feeling much more intense, "topping" others with even more aggression or wanting "to be fucked by lots of guys, as if I were worthless and being used by other people." Later, in therapy, he talked about more complicated feelings, such as relief: Brian had been afraid of getting HIV for so long that he actually felt liberated. He could have sex without worrying about getting HIV because he already had it. He considered the possibility that one of the reasons he had sex without condoms, in addition to the crystal high, was that he wanted to become HIV-positive—if he were positive, he thought, his experience of having sex wouldn't be plagued by the constant fear of catching HIV.

While smoking crystal and having sex with one man, Brian had a seizure. He does not recall what actually happened (typical of seizures), but he assumes that the man called 911 and fled his apartment—he was told by the hospital that the ambulance personnel found the door of his apartment open, and Brian lying naked and unconscious on the floor.

In therapy, Brian discussed how crystal helped him cope with the depression, fear, and anger he felt about getting HIV. It allowed him a brief relief from his sadness by elevating his mood, and it made him feel confident and powerful rather than frightened and powerless. While Brian believed some part of him may have wanted to get HIV, he also felt tremendous anger at himself for getting HIV, and he wanted to punish himself. In addiction, he felt angry in general—at HIV, at gay men, and at the world. The rough intensity of the sex was an outlet for his pent-up rage, wrapped in the deceptive guise of "hot sex."

Getting HIV, and his self-destructive binge, was a wake-up call for Brian. He considers himself lucky because he believes that many people he saw at sex parties or met online were in the same state of denial or self-destruction, but unlike him, they continued their behavior. Even though he ended up in the hospital, the humiliation of being found naked and unconscious by the ambulance team and possibly his neighbors, as well as the immediate possibility of dying, shook him awake: while HIV could possibly kill him if he did not start taking better care of himself, crystal was definitely putting him closer and closer to death.

CRYSTAL AND WOMEN—
WHAT ARE SPECIFIC ISSUES FOR FEMALES?

WHILE A SUBSTANTIAL number of women use or are addicted to meth, different studies find widely varying numbers. For example, in a meth study conducted by the University of California, San Diego (UCSD), only 24 percent of people responding to recruitment efforts were female, roughly one third the number of males. However, in another study from the University of California, Los Angeles (UCLA), which recruited subjects from a methamphetamine treatment center, females almost equaled males in number. Interpreting these data is difficult. In the UCSD study, it is not clear how and where potential subjects were solicited. If ads were placed in papers read more by men, or in places frequented more by men, then this could explain the dramatically greater number of men compared to women in the study. On the other hand, the UCLA study recruited subjects from a methamphetamine treatment center. Hypothetically, supposing women were more likely to seek help for addiction than men, the greater presence of women in that study would not accurately reflect the proportion of female to male meth addicts outside of treatment settings. The absolute number of women using meth remains unclear, but it is certain that many women use meth and do so with serious consequences.

Biologically, women's bodies handle crystal differently than men's. Women produce a form of the enzyme dopamine beta-hydroxylase that is slower than the form produced by men. This enzyme breaks down dopamine into adrenaline, which increases energy, elevates mood, and can also cause anxiety. It is likely that this difference results in gender-specific experiences of the drug. According to the UCLA study, the most common motivations to use crystal reported by women were to get high, to have fun, and to increase energy, which were similar motivations for men. However, there were also some significant differences. While improving energy was one of the most common reasons women reported, this was a much less frequent reason for men. While 14 percent of women reported using crystal to enhance sexual pleasure, 23 percent of men felt sex was an extremely important factor in their use. The most striking difference was that 36 percent of women identified weight loss as a reason they used meth, compared to only 7 percent of men. Clinically, we see the use of crystal for weight loss in drug rehabilitation programs and in hospital units treating women with severe anorexia and body-image disorders.

Though the UCLA study did not find sexual pleasure to be one of the primary motivations for women to use crystal, research consistently shows that using the drug while having sex intensified sexual pleasure in women similarly to how it has been reported by men. The powerful effect on sexual desire and behavior caused by crystal puts women at a higher risk of catching STDs or becoming pregnant.

Because meth can cause such intense hypersexuality, it can also be used as a date-rape drug. Usually we think of date-rape drugs as sedatives that make the victim mentally clouded or unconscious. With crystal, however, the victim remains wide awake and vibrantly clear. Because it stimulates sexual appetite so powerfully, the victim may be willing to have sex with almost anyone, including many people whom she would never even consider if she were sober. The drug changes her judgment so much that she is literally "not the same person," and she would pursue sex much more aggressively. It was likely she could also feel so compelled by sex that she might disregard her normal precautions and put herself at risk for STDs and pregnancy.

Given the hypersexual effects of crystal, unintended pregnancies are a considerable concern. Unfortunately, there are few studies examining how often this occurs. One study in Hawaii found that out of 546 deliveries, 1.4 percent of the babies tested positive for methamphetamine, which is a surprising figure considering that the general prevalence of meth use in the United States is 4.0 percent, and Hawaii is considered to have a significantly higher percentage of active meth users.

Crystal causes serious complications to both mothers and newborns. There have been numerous case reports of pregnant women using meth who came to the hospital with similar complications: premature delivery, preecclampsia/ecclampsia (dangerously high blood pressure before and during delivery), maternal cerebral hemorrhage (bleeding inside the mother's brain), and cardiovascular collapse (failure of the heart and circulatory system due to depleted dopamine and adrenaline) because mothers chronically exposed to meth were not able to tolerate anesthesia. In most of these cases, the mothers died.

Babies of meth-using mothers also suffered serious complications, including compromised placental blood flow (inadequate oxygen and nutrition to the developing fetus), premature delivery, low APGAR scores (poor color, breathing, and general responsiveness of the newborn at the time of delivery), and abnormal development of the baby's nervous system. Studies of rats exposed to meth during their gestation showed abnormal seizure activity, reflecting abnormal development of the surface of the brain.

Women must be aware that crystal's sexual effects can cause unplanned pregnancies, resulting in harm to the mother and child, with consequences as serious as death.

TEENS AND CRYSTAL—WHAT'S HOT AND WHAT'S NOT

THE 2002 NATIONAL Household Survey on Drug and Health reported that 1.5 percent of teenagers reported ever using crystal. Fortunately, this group has shown a slight decline in meth use—although very modest—in the past year. Adolescents have unique concerns about crystal use that should be known by teens, as well as parents, teachers, drug counselors, and policy makers.

Studies of teenagers in Taiwan, albeit culturally different from adolescents in the United States, can warn us of important issues that may also apply to teens in this country. Taiwanese studies showed that meth use in teens was associated with general behavioral problems; lower quality of caregiving, such as disrupted parental care and lower caregiver education; having adolescent peers who also use meth; and an alarmingly high rate of suicidal thoughts—16 percent—within the past year. Research at Duke University found that among American youth, recent meth users were more likely to be female, aged sixteen to seventeen years old. Use of meth in these teens was highly associated with criminal activity and recent problems with alcohol.

Research shows that adolescents have a pattern of using meth that is distinct from adults. It is associated with environmental factors that must be addressed, such as quality of parental care and the presence of meth in schools. In addition, teen-specific education about meth should be developed as a preventive measure—the fewer peers using meth, the lower the risk that a new teen will pick up the drug. With regard to depression, whether it is a cause for meth use or meth use results in more serious depression, teens should be carefully monitored for signs of problems with mood. Further studies hopefully will shed light on what aspects of crystal make it so much more appealing to female teens, whether it is the appetite-suppressing and weight-loss effect or another cultural or female-specific biological response to methamphetamine.

Last, there is mounting evidence that adolescent brains are particularly susceptible to damage from crystal. Brains continue developing in humans until early adulthood, so their reactions to drugs, as well as the damage that drugs cause, can differ greatly between adolescents and adults. Animal studies have already shown that adolescent brains exposed to methamphetamine show *more* structural damage than adult brains, particularly in areas such as the basal ganglia, and show greater deficits in cognition, meaning ability to think and learn. While human studies have shown the immediate problems associated with meth use in teens, animal studies have shown that teens who use meth may experience significant long-term problems with thinking, mood, behavior, and neurological disorders, such as Parkinson's disease.

CRYSTAL CAN AFFECT ANYONE: SOME SOBERING STATISTICS

THE APPEAL OF methamphetamine is broad because it is such a powerfully addictive drug. Once it gets a foothold in any community, its use spreads quickly, and significant numbers of people can be affected—in all age groups, ethnicities, religions, and sexual orientations. I gave detailed examples of two specific communities, gay men and heterosexual women, as illustrations of how particular groups can be affected. But the risk of meth addiction exists for people of any type, manifesting itself in different ways within each community.

Though there have been cycles of meth addiction in the past, this current wave is worse because of the rapid social changes in recent years, including growth of the Internet, greater ease of obtaining sex, and easily accessible information on how to make meth. Combined with other illnesses such as HIV and hepatitis B and C, we are currently witnessing an even greater public health disaster.

Despite U.S. government efforts to stem the rise of crystal use, it continues to increase and cause problems. According to the Drug Abuse Warning Network, the number of crystal-related emergency room visits increased from 10,447 in 1999 to 17,676 in 2002. The American Society of Addiction Medicine confirms this study and reports that states in the

Midwest are particularly affected: there, 70 to 80 percent of hospitals reported that meth was a factor in at least 10 percent of their patient visits. In addition, 47 percent of those midwestern hospitals surveyed identified crystal as the most common drug-related cause of emergency room visits. Some reasons included severe chemical burns of people trying to manufacture crystal, traumatic injuries linked to aggression, and paranoid behavior while high. Meanwhile, the demand for treatment of meth-related incidents or addiction has increased by 69 percent, causing a sharp rise in hospital costs; however, 63 percent of the hospitals also reported that they didn't have enough resources to meet the heavy demand for emergency care.

The initial concern about crystal and gay men was due to the increase in risky sexual behaviors. However, the preliminary findings of a study by the California Department of Health Services, Office of AIDS, show that sexual behavior of exclusively heterosexual men seems to follow the same pattern. Straight men using crystal, compared to a matched group of noncrystal-using straight men, were significantly more likely to be recently sexually active, have anal sex with women, have casual or anonymous sex, have multiple female sex partners, have sex with women who injected drugs, and have ever exchanged money or drugs for sex. Condom use did not differ much because its rate of use was generally low in all heterosexual men.

I STRONGLY EMPHASIZE that crystal can affect anybody. While there has been considerable media attention on crystal use in the gay male community because of its connection to HIV, gay men make up only a small minority of the total number of crystal users in the United States. This is extremely important to understand. The needs of all populations affected by crystal must be addressed, and funding for treatment services should be directed to all of the various communities. In addition, the recent tendency of many people to think of crystal as a gay drug may fuel homophobia and distract attention from the real problem of the potential dangers of crystal methamphetamine to all people.

2

WHAT EXACTLY IS CRYSTAL METHAMPHETAMINE?

METHAMPHETAMINE BELONGS TO a class of drugs called **stimulants**. Stimulants act on your brain in a way that increases alertness, and they work primarily on the neurotransmitter **dopamine**, as well as another chemical called **norepinephrine** (more commonly referred to as **adrenaline**). Dopamine is a chemical that affects not only your brain, but your heart, lungs, muscles, blood vessels, stomach, intestines, and even the blood vessels that line all the muscles and skin throughout your entire body. It has many functions depending on where it's acting. Methamphetamine is a very close cousin to amphetamine, differing only by the addition of a **methyl group**, a small cluster of atoms with a carbon atom and three hydrogen atoms.

Though the difference in the molecular structure is small, the effect that this small cluster of atoms has is tremendous, making methamphetamine the most powerful stimulant that exists. Other stimulants include amphetamine (sold under various brand names, such as Dexedrine and

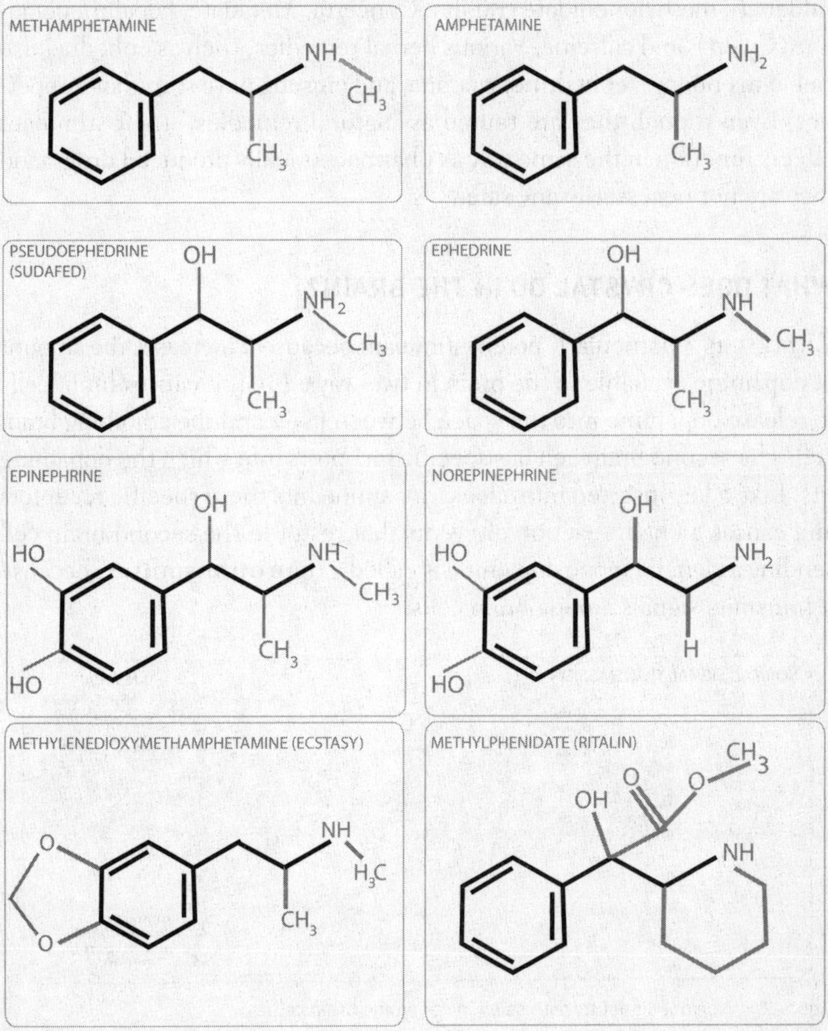

Figure 2-1. Chemical structure of methamphetamine and similar molecules.

Adderall), methylphenidate (Ritalin, Concerta, Metadate, Focalin), pemoline (Cylert), and caffeine. Various herbal remedies, such as ephedra (also called ma huang), ephedrine, guarana, and ginseng have stimulant properties. Even though they are touted as "natural remedies," their stimulant effects function in the same way as pharmaceutically produced drugs, and they are not necessarily any safer.

WHAT DOES CRYSTAL DO IN THE BRAIN?

CRYSTAL IS A particularly potent stimulant because it increases the amount of dopamine available to the brain in two ways: First, it causes brain cells to release dopamine into the space between itself and the adjoining brain cell. The second brain cell has specific receptors into which the dopamine fits. Like a key inserted into a lock, dopamine hits these specific receptors and causes a chain reaction of events that result in the second brain cell sending a signal. Hence dopamine is called a **neurotransmitter**, because it transmits signals among brain cells.

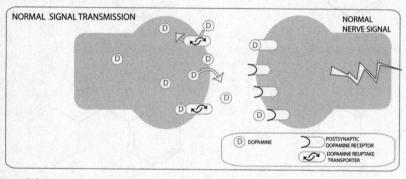

Figure 2-2. Normal signal transmission in dopamine brain cells.

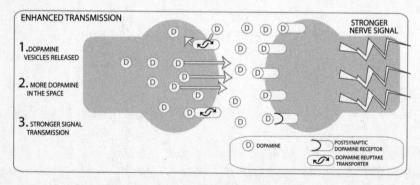

Figure 2-3. Signal transmission in dopamine brain cells with enhanced dopamine release.

The second action of methamphetamine is that it prevents the reuptake of dopamine back into the brain cell. In general, brain cells are good conservationists: they try to recycle neurotransmitters so that cellular energy isn't wasted on making large amounts of dopamine—the brain can simply reuse what it has already made. But meth blocks the recycling centers, called **dopamine transporters**, so that dopamine is trapped in the space between brain cells. Dopamine starts to accumulate, like water in a sink that's become clogged. The second brain cell is bombarded with more dopamine, and this results in increased stimulation of the cell and a much stronger signal transmission.

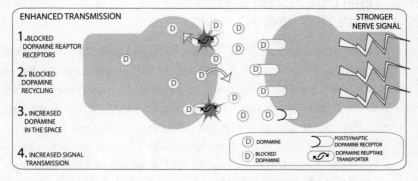

Figure 2-4. Signal transmission in dopamine brain cells with blocked reuptake.

Blocking dopamine reuptake is the primary way that cocaine works as a stimulant. Meth is much more powerful than cocaine because it does the same thing as cocaine, but it also causes an outpouring of dopamine, as shown in figure 2-3. Imagine a sponge, sopping wet with a fluid called dopamine. Crystal squeezes the sponge and grips it tightly, so that the sponge can't reabsorb any of the dopamine. The outpouring of dopamine when the saturated sponge is squeezed is the initial rush that meth users feel. This huge gush is also associated with the production of **free radicals**, chemically active particles that cause damage to the body. Free radicals have been implicated in causing genetic mutations, cancer, cell death, and aging. I will talk more about this in chapter 22.

When the brain has been flooded with dopamine that is unable to be recycled, the level of dopamine within the brain rises dramatically. In comparison to brains without any drug exposure, cocaine raises dopamine to levels 400 percent higher than normal. Methamphetamine is much more powerful and causes a 1,500 percent increase in dopamine. Clearly, this is far from the brain's natural state.

Although dopamine affects many parts of the brain and body, the effect most important to our discussion is upon the area called the ***nucleus accumbens***, which sends a dopamine-mediated signal to the ***ventral tegmentum***. These two brain sites connect by a bundle of brain cells called the **mesolimbic pathway**, or the "brain-reward circuit." This is one of the areas of the brain that is most powerfully associated with pleasure. However, it is also highly associated with addiction.

WHAT DOES USING CRYSTAL FEEL LIKE? IS IT REALLY THAT GOOD?

THE HUMAN BRAIN is made up of 20 to 50 billion cells. While the general arrangement of these cells is the same in all human brains, between individuals there are countless small differences in how these cells are arranged. Each experience you have and each new piece of information you learn causes small changes in the connections between brain cells. Also, anything you expose your body to, including food, drugs, and chemicals in the environment, has an impact on the way your brain develops. So each person's brain is unique. In addition, your body is unique in the way that your particular liver breaks down toxins, how easily your body stores drugs in fat cells, and how well it excretes drugs from your kidneys. Therefore, there is some variability in how each person experiences crystal, physiologically speaking. Nonetheless, there are some experiences that are common to most people, and in the following general description, the majority of people have *many* or *most* of the symptoms, though perhaps not *all*:

- Depending on *how* meth is taken, its effects can start almost immediately or may take a while. Swallowing methamphetamine or squirting it into the rectum can take 20 to 40 minutes to feel the effects. Snorting meth gives an effect in about 2 to 10 minutes. Smoking or injecting causes an effect almost immediately.
- People using meth often feel an initial rush of euphoria, followed by a strong sense of well-being and boosted self-confidence. Their moods are elevated, and if they were feeling depressed,

crystal may quickly lift them out of the blues and into an extremely happy state. Their senses are heightened, and sights and sounds may seem sharper and more vivid. On the other hand, just as if they have had too much coffee, some people may also feel jittery and anxious, or even panicky. In general, most people feel a tremendous boost of energy and confidence, believing that they can accomplish almost anything. People who were socially withdrawn suddenly are able to come out of their shells and see themselves as outgoing, charismatic personalities. Their brains work at a faster speed with more ideas coming to them. The boost in confidence makes these ideas seem brilliant, and there's a strong need to talk to others about these ideas, with people talking more and at a faster rate.

- Meth helps people to concentrate and do very focused activities. This can be great for the tired worker who has too many things to do and not enough time in the day to do them. This can be particularly dangerous because once people see themselves performing extraordinarily well, they may start to expect a level of work that's only possible by continuing to do more meth. Then working without the drug may seem slow, difficult, and relatively unproductive.

- When people use larger amounts of meth, their goal-directed behavior become extreme, resulting in the compulsive repetition of an activity. This could be a **stereotyped motor activity**, meaning repeating a single type of movement over and over again, such as rocking, chewing or grinding teeth, wringing hands, or fidgeting with objects. The behavior may extend to more complex activities, such as vigorously cleaning an entire house or searching in a purse for a ticket stub for 30 minutes. While the person is high, the activity makes sense, and there is a strong feeling of determination and purpose to the activity.

- In the extreme, the compulsive things people do on crystal are not productive. When they are sober, they may look back at what they've done, realizing that they've written volumes of nonsensical scribbling or spent hours rearranging a bookshelf that was already organized. But when they were high, their inflated confidence and strong determination tricked them into thinking that they were working on a brilliant project that made perfect sense at the time.

■ Like other stimulants, methamphetamine is an excellent appetite suppressant. People lose their appetite, and they may become so focused on some activity that they forget to eat at all. People have lost tremendous amounts of weight while doing crystal, though not in a healthy way. Rather, their bodies become malnourished, they lose healthy muscle, and they lack the vitamins and nutrients they need for optimal health.

■ Crystal can cause dry mouth and tooth grinding, and, along with malnutrition, it can also cause osteoporosis. When it is used frequently and for long periods of time, this combination of factors can result in severe dental problems, recently given the nickname **meth mouth**, that literally destroy teeth. The artificial boost in their self-esteem and the intense focus of attention on other things distracts crystal users, who may be completely unaware or unbothered by their dental decay.

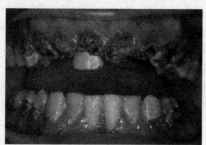

Figure 2-5. "Meth mouth." Photo taken by Michael I. Barr, DDS

■ In gay dance clubs and at circuit parties, crystal is becoming more and more the drug of choice, rather than Ecstasy or ketamine, which used to be the most popular drugs. Crystal helps people in these venues to dance longer and to feel more of the sexual energy of the pickup scene. Many partygoers feel a boost in self-confidence, which helps them feel sexier and more attractive, and so they behave more sexually aggressively than usual and have more courage to try to meet someone or proposition someone for sex. Fueled by the energy of crystal and the strong allure of a sexually charged environment, circuit partygoers are able to stay at marathon dance parties with little-to-no-sleep for several days. They become so involved in the dancing that they forget about all other activities, including eating, drinking, and, for those who have HIV, taking their medications, which depend on a strict time schedule. Alternatively, they may disregard the precautions they need to take for medications that they have already taken—combinations of meth with some medications, such as certain HIV medications, anti-infectious agents, and antidepressants, can be dangerous or even deadly. While users feel and think they look great, they may actually appear haggard and wasted. When the lights go on at the end of a club night, the sight of the last stragglers still dancing on crystal is not pretty.

■ Crystal users may disregard precautions concerning safer sex, or the quality of sex may be rougher, because they feel more aggressive and powerful, or they feel an insatiable hunger for sex. The intense need for sexual gratification often overshadows concerns about HIV, other sexually transmitted diseases, and pregnancy. For some, the excitement of playing with danger adds to the high.

WHAT HAPPENS IN YOUR BODY WHEN YOU USE CRYSTAL?

CRYSTAL WORKS PRIMARILY on dopamine, which has receptors not just in the brain but throughout the entire body. Dopamine is one of the chemicals that the body uses in the fight-or-flight response, which kicks in when one's brain senses there is an emergency or a threat to one's survival. Dopamine makes the heart beat harder and faster, and it constricts blood vessels in certain parts of the body, like the skin, nasal passages, and the intestines, so that blood can be redirected to other areas, such as muscles, which are more needed in a fight-or-flight situation. Blood pressure increases, and pupils dilate to let in more light and enable one to see a predator or an escape route better.

Here is a breakdown of what happens:

■ *The heart:* During this reaction, the heart is working overtime, meaning that it needs to have more oxygen (delivered to organs via the blood). However, high blood pressure can actually prevent blood from getting back to the heart because it makes it difficult to move blood through the vessels. In some cases, stimulants can cause blood vessels that feed the heart itself to constrict and prevent the heart from getting an adequate blood supply. This is what is called a heart attack, and it's possible that crystal users may suffer multiple tiny heart attacks over time, or more rarely, a large and serious one with obvious chest pain. Other symptoms of a heart in serious distress may include pain radiating from the chest to the jaw, left shoulder, or left arm; dizziness; shortness of breath; nausea; and vomiting, Any of these symptoms mean that someone should call 911 immediately, and the person should be taken directly to the emergency room.

- *The digestive system:* Because it is receiving less blood, the whole digestive tract slows down. This is one of the reasons that appetite decreases and bowel movements become less frequent. With extremely high doses of meth, the intestines can even suffer **bowel ischemia**, meaning that the muscles and lining of the intestines can die because of insufficient blood supply. Fortunately, this is rare.

- *The kidneys:* The kidneys filter all of the blood that flows through the body. The blood vessels and filtering units, called **nephrons**, are delicate and require a delicate balance of blood flow through them. They can be damaged by elevated blood pressure. However, they also require a minimum constant blood supply in order to stay alive. When people use crystal, they may initially have high blood pressure, but when they binge and do not drink fluids, they become dehydrated, and their blood pressure can become low, resulting in low blood flow to the kidneys. With an insufficient blood supply, kidney cells may die, and if there is enough damage, the kidneys may go into failure. People who use meth should remember to drink fluids regularly. If they are dancing in a hot room and sweating, they are losing even more water, and it's even more important to keep drinking liquids.

- *The muscles:* Crystal cranks up the whole body's system, and body temperature can become elevated. This, together with the several-day dance marathons of circuit parties, can increase the breakdown of muscle. Muscle breakdown products, such as **creatinine phosphokinase** (CPK), are toxic to the kidneys when they are present in high concentrations in the blood. This is another reason to keep drinking fluids to save one's kidneys—to dilute the toxic effects of CPK. When muscle breakdown is extreme, this is a condition called **rhabdomyolysis**, which can also damage kidneys and lead to kidney failure. People with rhabdomyolysis are usually given intravenous fluids to hydrate them as quickly as possible, dilute the toxic muscle breakdown products, and flush the toxins out. To avoid ever reaching that extreme state, remember to keep hydrated!

FOCUS ON CRYSTAL AND THE BRAIN: WHAT'S REALLY HAPPENING INSIDE YOUR HEAD

NUMEROUS STUDIES IN humans and in animals have shown that crystal causes changes in brain function and damages brain cells involved in dopamine and serotonin transmission. In particular, crystal decreased the function of brain cells in the **thalamus**, a central area that relays motor, sensory, and emotional signals to different parts of the brain; and the **striatum**, which deals with reward-linked motivation, planning, and impulse control. A study at the Brookhaven National Laboratory in Upton, New York, found that nine to eleven months after crystal users quit the drug, they were able to regain some activity in the thalamus, but the striatum remained impaired.

Some people argue that crystal does not "destroy" brain cells; however, several studies demonstrate that it damages *parts* of certain cells, some of them permanently. These cells can be compared to the long microfibers that carry telephone signals. If the ends of the microfibers are destroyed, the signal cannot reach its target. Similarly, even if an entire brain cell does not die, the destruction of just the end of the brain cell has profound effects on how well it is able to transmit the signal it is supposed to. Scientists nicknamed the effect of crystal on brain cells "pruning," meaning that the tips of affected brain cells are "cut off," much as a bush is pruned. Damaged brain cells try to compensate by sprouting new branches, but studies show that the function remains impaired.

Functional imaging of the brain with **PET (positron emission tomography) scans** shows what parts of the brain are active during different activities, such as resting, concentrating, or thinking different emotional thoughts. These imaging studies have consistently shown differences in the way that the brains of heavy crystal users function compared to brains that have never been exposed to the drug. These differences are in areas that use dopamine, as well as glutamate, which is used in the frontal cortex. Recent studies show that longtime stimulant users may be more prone to **Parkinson's disease** and other movement disorders, which are related to damage in areas of the brain that function with dopamine.

Supporting the data from PET scans, studies that directly test the mental function of heavy crystal users compared to nonusers show that the former group demonstrate impaired mental function, particularly complex thinking that involves adapting to changing situations, various aspects of memory, weighing judgments, and decision making. Unfortunately, *these are areas of thinking that you must use to keep yourself from falling back into drug use*. Without these faculties, it is much more difficult for an addict to fight off relapses. Continued crystal use literally changes the brain so that it becomes harder to mentally resist the urge to keep using.

Recently, research has found that the meth-related damage to **serotonin** neurons is associated with less control of aggression and impulses. If these functions are weakened, then an addict's ability to resist the temptation of using a drug again is even harder. In even more ways, the brain becomes hard-wired to keep itself on crystal.

WHAT HAPPENS IF YOU TAKE TOO MUCH CRYSTAL?

STIMULANT TOXICITY IS common with regular users. What is it like when someone uses too much crystal?

- Anxiety and difficulty sleeping are common, even with lower doses and infrequent use.
- Rather than euphoria or positive mood, some people experience agitation, irritability, and impatience.
- With a tremendous strain on the heart, crystal can cause heart attacks, which can be small and painless or significant, with tremendous chest pain or even death.
- The increase in brain activity can cause seizures in some people, especially if they have a history of seizures or are simultaneously taking other drugs or medications that increase seizure risk.
- With high doses and frequent or regular use, people can become paranoid, feeling that they are being followed or watched. They

may start keeping the shades drawn and react to small noises, fearful that someone is following or harassing them. Paranoia can become quite elaborate, with beliefs that the CIA or neighbors are following them. They can start to have hallucinations—hearing voices, seeing things, and feeling sensations such as bugs crawling on their skin. The reason for these symptoms is overstimulation of the dopamine system in the brain. Too much dopamine is one of the brain malfunctions in schizophrenia, and the behavior of people with severe stimulant toxicity can mimic that of paranoid schizophrenics. Many meth users have been admitted to psychiatric hospitals and treated with medications for schizophrenia because the symptoms appear identical.

■ There is a "kindling" effect with stimulant psychosis, meaning that the more a person experiences psychotic symptoms, such as paranoia and hallucinations, the greater is the likelihood of experiencing psychosis the next time he or she uses meth, and the psychosis can become increasingly severe and last longer, even days to weeks after the person stops using crystal.

HOW IS CRYSTAL MADE?

CRYSTAL IS RELATIVELY easy to make. Early methods were based on recipes using phenyl-2-propanone, mercuric acid, aluminum foil, and methylamine. More recent production methods are simpler, made with over-the-counter cold remedies, such as the nasal decongestant Sudafed (**pseudoephedrine**), and lithium from rechargeable batteries.

While some of the ingredients, such as pseudoephedrine, are safe, many of the ingredients are extremely toxic: mercury, aluminum, **anhydrous ammonia** (commonly used by farmers as fertilizer), **toluene** (a solvent used in paint, glue, and gasoline), **methanol** (an extremely toxic form of alcohol used in industrial processing), **ether** (one of the first chemicals used for surgical general anesthesia), lye, **muriatic acid** (concentrated hydrochloric acid, used to clean mortar and brick), iodine, and rubbing alcohol. These ingredients are mixed and heated, and elements are extracted to form methamphetamine.

In addition to problems associated methamphetamine itself, there are dangers of using street meth because it is unlikely to be pure. Some of the toxic agents listed above may not have been fully processed, and may therefore still be in their original form in what is sold on the street. In particular, mercury, methylene, and aluminum are well known to cause serious medical problems, such as brain injury and damage to the brain, liver, and kidneys.

Crystal has been produced in thousands of small basement labs throughout the country, particularly in rural areas, where the strong, noxious smells and the potentially explosive reactions attract less attention. Recently, the federal and local governments have been clamping down on meth labs, closing down 17,000 labs in 2002 alone. In addition, many localities have been passing legislation to limit the supply of such ingredients as nasal decongestants, making them more difficult to buy in any significant quantity. During this recent period, production has shifted to "superlabs" outside the United States, to countries where supplies are easier to obtain and production can continue with less interference from law enforcement. The U.S. Drug Enforcement Agency estimates that 80 percent of all methamphetamine used by Americans is produced in Mexico. Still, thousands of small basement labs within the United States are continuing to produce crystal from recipes that are readily available on the Internet.

A particular danger of online recipes is that they are not regulated or reviewed by anyone to guarantee their authenticity or accuracy. And many of the recipes are crude, so even when they are correct, they are likely to leave many contaminants and unprocessed toxic chemicals in the final product.

Here is an unedited excerpt from a Web page of one "basement" manufacturer, describing how he makes meth:

> Shake the jars till pills are completely broke down, then let the jars sit again for 4 hours or until the Heats is completely clear. Once clear cyphon the heat off (Not the powder stuff at the Bottom you don't want this it will fuck your dope up). Well anyways syphon the hear off with a piece of the sergical tubing syphon this into a pyrodex baking dish...if it's this color you have done good at cooking the dope now to add colemans fuel fill the far full just anough room for shaking now add 1-2 teaspoons of red devil lye let the jar site aofr about 5 mins then place lid on the jar and shake the hell out of it.
>
> —http://totsei.com, accessed April 12, 2005

The writer seems marginally literate and unsophisticated, yet he is handling dangerous chemicals. The recipe is crude and filled with potential for mistakes that could allow the final product to contain chemicals far more toxic than methamphetamine. But his incoherence notwithstanding, the mixture described above has likely been snorted, smoked into the lungs, or injected directly into the bloodstream of many unfortunate people.

The impurity of crystal is not just a frightening supposition. A 2003 study of methamphetamine, released by the White House Office of Drug Control Policy, reported that from 1994 to 2001, the average purity of methamphetamine found in the United States had decreased from 71.9 to 40.1 percent. That means that of the crystal that you buy on the street, *up to 60 percent* is not methamphetamine—rather, it could contain fillers, other drugs you never intended to take, and toxic leftovers from the production process.

At the time of this writing, several states and municipalities have passed laws to limit the availability of pseudoephedrine to any single individual. Since then, domestic production in basement labs has dramatically decreased, and the majority of manufacturing has shifted to Mexico. Despite production in Mexican superlabs, which churn out large volumes at a rapid pace, "factory-produced" crystal is not necessarily any safer than basement-brand crystal. There are no restrictions or guidelines on the production of methamphetamine in these illegal superlabs. Recent reports indicate that the purity of crystal produced in superlabs is indeed higher, but the unexpected and the unpredictable increase in potency has resulted in a number of overdoses, ER visits, and deaths.

Consider this cautionary reminder: In 2004, there was a health alert concerning children who may have eaten certain candies produced in Mexico that contained chili or tamarind. Because of poor regulation of these *legal* products, it was found that many of the candies, which had been exported to American markets, contained dangerous levels of lead, and thus children who ingested the candies may have suffered lead poisoning. Imagine how much less controlled foreign factory production of *illegal* substances is. *Let the buyer beware.*

UNDERSTANDING ADDICTION:
What Is It and Do You Have It?

STRATEGY:
Take a Close Look at the Role
Crystal Plays in Your Life

Objectives:
- Learn precisely what addiction is.
- Learn the distinct attributes of crystal that make it so addictive.
- Learn about the many uses of crystal besides just getting high. Is it really just a recreational, fun activity, or is it a crutch that helps with other needs?
- Carefully examine your use of crystal to see if it fits the pattern of addiction.

MEDICAL DISEASE OR WEAK PERSONALITY? WHAT IS ADDICTION?

BEFORE DISCUSSING THE addictive properties of crystal, it is important to under-
stand the concept of **addiction** itself. "Addiction" is difficult to define
because the term is used so commonly in the English language. The word
is casually used in such situations as "I'm addicted to soap operas," or
"I'm addicted to chocolate." Even among different medical specialties,
there is disagreement about how exactly to define addiction.

The Diagnostic and Statistical Manual of Mental Disorders, Fourth
Edition (DSM-IV), a diagnostic reference book published by the American
Psychiatric Association (APA), uses the term "substance dependence" to
define drug addiction. Using this new term with its specific definition
avoids the confusion of all the different meanings that "addiction" has. In
this book, the word "addiction" refers to the APA definition of substance
dependence.

In essence, DSM-IV defines substance dependence as a pattern of continued use of any substance despite the fact that it has become harmful to
the person using it. This means that even though a drug causes problems

in a person's health, daily function, or other important aspects of life, the addict is unable to stop using it.

The fundamental concept of substance dependence is that a person no longer has *control* of the drug or the use of it—rather, the drug is controlling the person, whether by psychological or physiological means. Despite the growing problems the drug creates, the addict continues to use or increase the amount and frequency of use.

"Loss of control" does not necessarily mean that an addict is *aware* of any problem—this is a major reason addicts allow drug use to increase to such an unhealthy extreme. The longer a drug is used, the more distorted the drug user's judgment becomes, and behavior that would never have been acceptable now becomes tolerable if it is necessary to allow the addict to keep using the drug.

For example, a successful attorney who had a perfect attendance record at the office, often working later than her colleagues, starts occasionally blowing off steam on Friday nights by doing a couple of bumps of crystal. Eventually her Friday routines regularly include doing meth, then going to bars to pick up men for casual sex. Over a few years, with increasingly longer and frequent crystal binges, she gradually finds herself calling in sick on Mondays because of crashing from weekend-long binges She doesn't question it because she feels that she had always overworked, and she believes that giving herself this enjoyment in life is a much smarter way to live.

In another example, a teenager who was always a model student tries meth so that she can study longer hours for her exams. She starts using it regularly to get her work done and gets hooked. Like most teens addicted to crystal, she eventually stealing. Having no job and only a small allowance from her parents, she secretly pawns valuables from her home so she can buy more meth, even though in her precrystal days, she would never have imagined herself stealing from her family.

DSM-IV DEFINITION OF SUBSTANCE DEPENDENCE

SUBSTANCE DEPENDENCE: A maladaptive pattern of substance use, leading to clinically significant impairment or distress, as manifested by three (or more) of the following, occurring at any time in the same 12-month period:

1. Tolerance, as defined by either of the following:
   a. A need for markedly increased amounts of the substance to achieve intoxication or desired effect.
   b. Markedly diminished effect with continued use of the same amount of the substance.
2. Withdrawal, as manifested by either of the following:
   a. The characteristic withdrawal syndrome for the substance.
   b. The same (or a closely related) substance is taken to relieve or avoid withdrawal symptoms.
3. The substance is often taken in larger amounts or over a longer period than was intended.
4. There is a persistent desire or unsuccessful efforts to cut down or control substance use.
5. A great deal of time is spent in activities necessary to obtain the substance (e.g., visiting several doctors or driving long distances), use the substance (e.g., chain-smoking), or recover from its effects.
6. Important social, occupational, or recreational activities are given up or reduced because of substance use.
7. The substance use is continued despite knowledge of having a persistent or recurrent physical or psychological problem that is likely to have been caused or exacerbated by the substance (e.g., current alcohol use despite recognition that an ulcer was made worse by alcohol).

Reprinted with permission from the Diagnostic and Statistical Manual of Mental Disorders, Fourth Edition, Text Revision Copyright 2000. American Psychiatric Association.

In practical terms, the DSM-IV breaks down addiction into three broad areas:

The first is a physiological adjustment of the body so that it needs more of the drug. This is either apparent by needing to use more to get the same amount of a high, or feeling terrible when the drug is stopped, because your body needs the drug in its system just to feel normal. The terrible feeling of withdrawal is what keeps many people continuing to use, even when they are not pursuing a high.

The second concept covered by the definition of substance dependence is that the space it takes up in your life grows larger and larger. You gradually use more of the drug, you spend more time and money using it, and you find yourself going to great lengths to get it. Its importance grows to the point that it outweighs other things in your life, and when given the choice between the drug and other pleasurable or important activities, such as spending time with friends or family, meeting deadlines, or doing your job properly, the drug seems increasingly attractive.

The drug becomes so important that you end up going to great lengths to get it, finding yourself doing things that you ordinarily wouldn't: spending money that should have been used for paying bills; going to dangerous neighborhoods or inviting dangerous people into your home, to buy drugs from a dealer; going to many different doctors, feigning illnesses and symptoms to get more prescription pills. Before becoming addicted, someone might never have done these things, but once addiction sets in, putting oneself at risk, shirking responsibilities, avoiding loved ones, and lying seems trivial compared to the need to use more drugs.

The third concept is loss of control. The physiological or psychological need for the drug becomes a monster, though this may develop so gradually it goes unnoticed. Over time, a drug user may spend less time with friends and family and more time with other people. But as addiction sets in and becomes stronger, even worse things happen, and the addict takes greater risks while using drugs, becoming estranged from family and friends, developing health problems directly related to drug use, engaging in unsafe activities while being high, dropping or flunking out of school, or losing a job. Despite these negative consequences of drug use, the addict cannot stop. Loss of control can be so complete that it may seem that the addict has even lost control of logical thinking. For example, a heavy crystal user may find that even though he knows that his drug use is causing him to feel paranoid and fearful, he does not want to stop. In the past he would never have let his life deteriorate to such a low, but addiction hijacks the brain and now it seems he does not even care about the frightening paranoia—the most important thing in the world is doing more drugs.

5

WHAT IS ALL THE HYPE
ABOUT CRYSTAL?

Is It Really More Addictive Than Other Drugs?

FIRST, A FEW BASICS ABOUT HOW THE BRAIN WORKS:
BRAIN FUNCTION 101

AS MENTIONED EARLIER, deep in the brain lies a bundle of neurons (brain cells) called the mesolimbic pathway, or the "brain-reward circuit." This bundle travels from an area in the brainstem called the ventral tegmentum to another area called the nucleus accumbens. This deep brain structure is nicknamed the "primitive brain" because it is shared by most animals and developed early in the evolution of species. All things that are vital to living are controlled by the primitive brain. This brain area controls your breathing, maintains your heartbeat, and tells you when it is time to eat, sleep, and wake up. It also controls behaviors such as eating and sex, of which we are aware and over which we have some limited control. The primitive brain functions are very powerful and difficult to override. For example, if you try to stop breathing, assuming you don't give up from sheer distress, you eventually pass out, lose consciousness, and start breathing again. The primitive brains wins. Similarly, if you fly from New York to London, your primitive brain is still functioning on New York time. Even if you know it's morning in London and you have to wake up, your primitive brains insists that it's still nighttime, and it's a struggle to feel fully alert. This phenomenon, commonly called "jetlag," is an example of the primacy of the primitive brain.

The brain-reward circuit, which lies in the primitive brain, is Mother Nature's way of tricking animals to repeat behaviors that are important for the long-term survival of the species. In the evolutionary model, behaviors that help an animal to live and have offspring are the most important because they help the entire species to survive. Therefore, activities such as eating and sex are tied to the brain-reward circuit. The species would eventually die out without eating or having sex. They are activities that most creatures do with pleasure, and there is a "compulsive" need to eat and have sex repeatedly. In this manner, the brain-reward circuit has helped humans, as well as most other species, to survive.

Humans also have a higher, more sophisticated part of the brain that developed much later in evolution: the wrinkled outer part of the brain called the **neocortex** (meaning "newly-developed cover"). This is where complex rational thinking occurs. The neocortex in humans is more developed than the cerebral cortex of any other species. The wrinkles on the outside of the human brain developed because there was not enough room on the surface of the primitive brain to accommodate the growing cortex, so as it continued to grow, it folded over itself, creating wrinkles, which are called sulci. The human brain, with its highly evolved cortex, is what gives us much higher powers of reasoning and logic compared to other animals. This is the part of the brain that is rational and tells overweight people, "You need to lose weight, so you should stop eating so much." However, control centers for appetite and the drive to eat do not reside in the cerebral cortex. They are in the primitive brain. This is one of the reasons that it is so difficult to diet, despite the intellectual knowledge that obesity is unhealthy—there is a constant struggle between the deeper brain and the logical cortex.. As in the example of trying to hold your breath and stop breathing, usually the deep brain wins.

This does *not* mean that it is *impossible* to overcome the deep brain impulses. There are many success stories of people who overcame obesity and lost impressive amounts of weight through diet and exercise. However, the work is hard, as most success stories will attest. The battle between the logical cortex and the primitive brain is a tough one.

ADDICTION IN THE BRAIN:
YES, THERE IS A MEDICAL REASON FOR IT

ALL DRUGS THAT are addictive somehow affect the brain-reward circuit. The more directly they tie into this circuit, the more they cause compulsive, uncontrollable use of the drug. Alcohol, nicotine, heroin, marijuana, cocaine, and methamphetamine all stimulate this pathway to some extent. Because the brain-reward circuit sends its signals via dopamine, drugs that increase the release of dopamine in this part of the brain are more addictive. Cocaine and methamphetamine are powerful dopamine-enhancing drugs, methamphetamine being the more powerful of the two.

The more often a drug stimulates the brain-reward circuit, the primitive brain becomes more strongly programmed to repeat the behavior of using that drug. Even months or years after stopping crystal use, people can still have strong urges to use. Even after years of abstinence, when the craving has been reduced to almost negligible thoughts, a small psychological trigger, such as a familiar place or situation, or a small exposure to the drug is all it takes to bring back the intensity of the compelling urge that has been programmed into the brain.

The neurochemistry of addiction is still a new field, and scientists are continually learning more about how the brain works during drug use and during the craving that pulls people back to using the drug again. In addition to dopamine, other parts of the brain are involved, such as the surface of the front of the brain called the prefrontal cortex. Communication between this area and the brain-reward circuit, as well as other areas, determines behavior—how someone feels when exposed to a reminder of a drug and how he or she makes a decision about what to do next (e.g., to go ahead and use the drug or to move along and do something else). This process is mediated by a chemical called **glutamate**. Recent studies reveal that addictive drugs, and in particular methamphetamine, cause destruction of brain cells that mediate these glutamate signals, and after that happens the signals do not work properly. Therefore, even if a person rationally knows that crystal has been destructive to his or her life, the brain has less of an ability to take this information and translate it into rational behavior: it becomes much harder to resist doing the drug again.

THE PSYCHOLOGICAL ASPECT OF ADDICTION: WHEN DRUGS ARE USED AS A CRUTCH

THE BRAIN-REWARD pathway is one of many causes of addiction. Another is the psychological relief that some drugs provide for emotional difficulties, such as anxiety. Crystal in particular can be a crutch for many different problems, such as depression, low self-esteem, fatigue, boredom, and difficulty working long hours. It also decreases appetite in order to lose weight. Most assume that people use drugs to feel high and to take them away from reality. However, some people suffer so much from other emotional struggles that drugs help treat the pain and "bring them back to center," making them feel more "normal." For some people, drugs are a way that they have found to deal with the reality of day-to-day living.

While stimulants are particularly good at enhancing low mood, "downers," in contrast, such as alcohol, heroin, ketamine, and certain prescription pills, such as Valium, Xanax, and OxyContin, can help with anxiety, provide an "escape" from troublesome thoughts and feelings, or numb emotional pain. This is an important concept to understand in drug treatment.

The take-home point here is that whatever drugs someone abuses, he or she should think about what kind of difficult feelings the drugs might be covering up. If there is a better way to cope, the drugs may not be so necessary.

Whatever the reason is that you may have started using a drug, after using it regularly to obtain emotional relief, your mind and your brain both become accustomed to a "quick fix." There is an AA expression, "Hold your belly," which encourages people to "stop your bellyaching and complaining." This is not a cold and unsympathetic statement—it is a reminder that you can tolerate some degree of frustration or uncomfortable feeling without going straight to a drug to make it instantly disappear. "Hold your belly" for a short time and let yourself sit with the feeling. Relearn that you do not need the quick fix and that all problems do not need to be fixed or erased immediately. The strong need for immediate gratification and a low tolerance for frustration are two psychological features that usually develop in most drug addicts. Remember that you can survive if you wait a little or take the longer, more productive route to address a problem, and that, if you do something other than use drugs, you may be able to do more than hide from the problem for a few hours—you may even fix it!

SOME SPECIFIC PSYCHOLOGICAL CONSIDERATIONS FOR GAY MEN

CRYSTAL may be particularly helpful with sexuality issues for gay men because of internalized feelings that being gay is bad. Even those who are completely "out and proud" may have deeply hidden notions that homosexuality is shameful. People have a tendency to internalize the values of their parents and their community, even when they intellectually disagree with them. A common example that illustrates the process of unconscious internalization is a young boy who is angry at his parents and says, "I'll never be like them when I grow up! I can't believe they treat me this way!" However, when the boy grows older, he observes his own behavior and remarks with surprise, "Oh my God, I'm turning into my father!"

Gay males have a natural attraction to other males, and they experience pleasure engaging in sex with other men. Yet, at the same time, they grew up in a society that to a great extent still labels homosexuality morally bad and socially repugnant. Therefore having gay sex can be like wandering through a flowery field filled with landmines. On the surface it looks as if it should be easily enjoyable, but it is full of hidden emotional bombs that complicate sex with feelings of guilt and self-hatred. When a man's biological urge to be with other men is criticized by both the internal voices and the external attitudes of society, the result is ambivalence, confusion, and anxiety about having sex. The intense hypersexuality of meth provides gay men an experience of *unconflicted*, unbridled sexual passion that many gay men have never experienced. Perhaps this is one reason why the gay male community has been particularly affected by crystal.

WHEN YOUR BODY NEEDS A DRUG JUST TO FEEL NORMAL: PHYSICAL DEPENDENCE IN ADDICTION

A THIRD ASPECT of addiction is physical dependence on a drug. Heavy drinkers who consume alcohol daily know the feeling of edginess, anxiety, and tremors that occur if they stop drinking for more than one or two days. Heroin addicts know the feeling of aches, chills, sweats, and intense emotional misery when they stop using heroin.

Crystal can cause an acute withdrawal, with fatigue, hunger, increased but irregular sleep, and depression that is sometimes so intense that people feel suicidal. Fear of the crash is what keeps some people using continually, and it becomes less about chasing the high and more about running away from the impending low. Depression and fatigue from a crash are most noticeable during the first seven to fourteen days after stopping crystal. Beyond that point, most people feel "back to normal," though the brain is actually still not working up to its baseline level. After heavy and regular use of crystal, it may take six to twenty-four months for someone's brain to reach a level of function close to how it had worked before that person ever used crystal.

DO YOU THINK
YOU MAY BE ADDICTED?

IF YOU USE crystal methamphetamine, how do you know if you are addicted? Not every user becomes an addict, and of those who do, the time it takes to develop an addiction varies. Some people are hooked immediately, and after just one try, they feel so amazingly good that they know that have to use more. However, for the vast majority of users, losing control of crystal is a gradual process that is so subtle, it goes unnoticed until it is too late. This more common experience of a slow development of addiction is consistent with the current understanding of brain physiology. Each exposure to crystal may cause a small but lasting change in the circuitry and function of brain cells. After enough exposures, the neuronal pattern changes enough and the user crosses a threshold where he or she can no longer resist the temptation to use crystal. The brain pathways that mediate decision making have become set so that using crystal is priority number one, regardless of what other parts of the brain logically think or desire.

So how does this translate into practical terms? In general, addiction means loss of control, but knowing when one has lost control can be difficult to discern. There are several ways to assess whether you have a problem with controlling crystal in your life. The "CAGE questionnaire," developed in 1974 as a medical screening tool, has become a favorite of general practice physicians who screen their patients for addiction. It is a simple screening tool with the following four questions:

C: Have you ever tried to Cut down on your drug use?
A: Are you ever Annoyed when people mention your drug use?
G: Do you ever feel Guilty about your drug use?
E: Do ever you use drugs first thing in the morning (an "Eye-opener")?

If you answer yes to two or more questions, there is a very good chance that you have a substance-use problem. The CAGE questionnaire was originally designed to screen for alcoholism, and it has been scientifically validated and found to pick up approximately 93 percent of people with alcohol dependency. Because of its high sensitivity and studies that demonstrate its usefulness in different scenarios, the CAGE questionnaire has been used to screen for addictions to other drugs, such as crystal methamphetamine.

In addition to the CAGE questionnaire, here are some additional questions to ask yourself to help examine your drug use and level of control:

1. *How often do you use crystal and has your use been increasing?* Do you use crystal once every few months, only when someone offers it to you? Did you start out this way, but gradually your use has increased to every other weekend? Did you plan the increase in use or did it sneak up on you? Has your use increased to *every* weekend, and do you find that you can't wait for the work week to end so you can use crystal again? Are you using crystal every day?

2. *How much crystal do you use?* Do you only have one bump, and then you're good for the rest of the night? Have you increased to doing several bumps or snorting lines? Are you able to do a bump and then put the bag away and leave it alone until another day, or do you usually have to go back for more? Have you noticed that the amount that used to get you high is no longer enough, and you now need much more?

3. *How much money do you spend on crystal?* Has the amount been increasing? Have you ever been in a situation where you did not have enough money but somehow had to scramble for the cash by borrowing money, going into credit card debt, leaving bills unpaid, or selling things in order to pay for crystal?

4. *How do you use crystal?* Has this changed over time? Did you start out snorting crystal, but later you started trying new ways to get a better or more intense high, such as smoking or slamming, or booty bumping?

5. *Where are you using crystal?* Are you using crystal only at rare social events? Has crystal become less of a social drug, and now you find yourself using it alone? Has crystal become more of a solitary activity except for sexual hookups? Have you become more isolated, seeing fewer of your friends and family because you are too busy using crystal?

6. *Have you ever had health problems somehow related to crystal?* This could include:
   a. Chest pains that felt like you might be having a heart attack
   b. Catching a sexually transmitted disease because you were having sex while high and not taking your usual safety precautions to protect yourself
   c. Becoming pregnant because you felt so driven to have sex while you were high that you didn't care that you weren't using contraceptives
   d. Panic attacks
   e. Depression, anxiety, or suicidal thoughts after you stopped using
   f. Psychotic symptoms, such as paranoia that people were watching you or eavesdropping, feeling that there was a plot against you, hearing voices or seeing things, or feeling sensations like bugs crawling on your skin
   g. Dental problems from dry mouth, tooth grinding, and neglecting your teeth
   h. For people with HIV, finding that your CD4 count or viral load has been worsening, or having difficulty adhering to your medication regimen because you were too busy partying

If you answered yes to any of the above or have had any other health problems related to crystal use, did you use crystal again, even after realizing that crystal caused these problems?

7. *Have you ever had trouble with your job because of crystal use?* Were you ever late for work or had to call in sick because you could not stop partying over the weekend, or when you did stop, you felt too bad from the crash to work? Did your job performance ever suffer? Did you ever get fired because of poor job performance or poor job attendance due to crystal? Did you still use crystal, even though you saw it affecting your work and possibly threatening your livelihood?

8. *Have you found yourself doing things to get crystal that you would never have done in the past?* Have you invited drug dealers who were unsavory or potentially dangerous people into your home, or have you gone to dangerous places to get crystal?

9. *Do you find that crystal determines the people you spend your time with?* Would you be spending time with the same people if you didn't share the bond of using crystal. Have you invited people into your life that the old you would never have considered as possible friends? Have you been spending less time with important people in your life who don't use drugs?

10. *Is crystal a "take-it-or-leave-it" option, or has it grown into a requirement?* Did it begin as an occasional fun treat at social activities but gradually became something you *needed* to enjoy yourself? Is it something that helps you get through a rare (two or three times a year) day of hard work, or has it turned into something you frequently use to do your job? Is it an occasional "extra spice" you add during sex, or has it become a requirement for sex to feel satisfying? Is crystal an option or a necessity?

11. *Has the number of reasons you use crystal multiplied?* Perhaps you started out using it just to have fun at special parties, but you found more and more reasons or excuses to use it: it makes things more fun, it makes you more confident, sex is much better, it's great to celebrate happy events, it's a lifesaver that rescues you from a sad mood, it helps you when you're bored. Gradually, crystal has become the "drug of all seasons," appropriate for any occasion. Do you always have an excuse to justify using?

These questions are a good way for you to stop and closely examine how you use crystal and how your use may have changed over time. If your pattern has changed and grown over time while you have been blind to it, you likely are developing an addiction.

WHAT IF I'M STILL NOT SURE?

IF YOU'VE GONE through this list of questions and you recognize that your crystal use has changed over time and grown, but you are still unsure if you are really addicted, the following exercises may help you check your level of control:

EXERCISE 6-1 STOP USING CRYSTAL COMPLETELY FOR ONE MONTH, STARTING TODAY

FIRST, take a good look at your response to reading this challenge. Did you feel that it would be no problem? Was your first reaction a sudden pang of fear that it would be difficult? Like many people, did you think this exercise would be no problem, but you didn't want to stop *today* because there was a special event coming up or you had already planned a special weekend or just bought a bag from your dealer? The last reaction, probably the most common, is a sign that you are rationalizing, telling yourself that you have control, though "now is just not a good time." For an addict, despite any plans to stop someday in the future, there is *never* a good time to quit. If you truly do not need crystal, then you can make it through any "special event" or difficult time without it. You should be able to commit to this exercise and say with conviction, "Yes, I can quit drugs for one month starting *right now*," and you should be able to follow through on your commitment.

EXERCISE 6-2 MAKE A CONTRACT WITH YOURSELF
FOR THE NEXT SIX MONTHS

WHEN you are sober, on a piece of paper, make a six-month plan by answering the following questions:

1. On how many occasions do you plan to use crystal during the next six months (how many total occasions in the next six months, or how occasions per month)?
2. How long do you plan to use crystal on each occasion? Just a quick bump to kick off a night out with friends, several bumps spread over the course of a night, or a three-day "weekend warrior" event at a circuit party or on vacation?
3. How much crystal will you use on each occasion and how much money is a reasonable limit to spend during each month of the entire six-month period?
4. In what situations are you going to use crystal? Only at parties, while hanging out with friends, at sex clubs, or at home alone?
5. How you are going to use crystal? Snorting only, smoking, slamming, booty bumping?

Answer these five questions on paper as specifically as you can, making these the upper limits of what you plan to use over the next six months. The upper limit should be similar to what your current use is, or if you'd like to cut down, what you think is a smaller but reasonable amount to use. Do not set limits that are *more* than your current use because this is like planning to be "out of control."

Next to each item, leave an empty checkbox. At the bottom of the paper, write:

I, [write your name], make a solemn commitment to myself to use crystal according to the above guidelines until six months from today's date. These guidelines were written by me, of my own free will. In my current state of mind, I believe these are reasonable limits to using crystal. With this in consideration, I understand that exceeding the limits, in any way and for whatever reason, indicates that I am not able to control my use.

Sign and date the paper, make a copy, put each copy in separate sealed envelopes, give one copy to a trusted friend, and keep one for yourself. On your calendar, mark the date six months ahead, and over the next six months, keep track of the information you outlined in the contract.

On the appointed day in six months, open the envelope and see how you did. Take a look at your reaction to how you did, as well as whether you think your guidelines from six months ago still seem reasonable. If you were able to stick to your limit or remain below it, congratulations! You may still have some control over your crystal use. To make sure that you maintain control, I strongly suggest repeating this contract every six months to keep track of your use to make sure that it continues to be in your control.

Some people find that they exceeded their maximum limit, but they don't mind. Despite the clause "in any way and for whatever reason," they feel justified in breaking the contract, giving excuses such as unforeseen "special circumstances." This demonstrates how reasons to use insidiously multiply, and addiction constantly searches for ways to trick the mind into using more. Addiction works silently in the brain, and even though these people can't keep their meth use within their own self-determined limits, they cannot see any problem.

Some find that their perspectives have changed over the six-month period, and they decide that they grossly underestimated how much crystal would be enough—they believe that they must not have been thinking clearly when they wrote the contract. However, they wrote the contract when they were in a distinctly clear and sober mental state. Something in their minds is now different, and more crystal is now acceptable. This change is the process of addiction. While the person may be unaware of any changes from six months prior, his or her need for crystal has grown, and to accommodate the increased need, the person's perception of what is acceptable has changed, as well.

Some people who were unable to stick to their contracts can clearly see that crystal use is not in their control. They are fortunate because this rapid insight is rare, and it can be a powerful tool that can be used to overcome the addiction if they are motivated to stop.

If you exceeded the limits *that you set for yourself*, regardless of the reason, there is no acceptable excuse. If you broke the contract, you do not have control. You broke a contract that nobody forced you into. Nobody made any unreasonable demands. You set your own "fair" ground rules. *If you cannot even follow your own wishes, then clearly you are not controlling yourself–crystal is.*

EXERCISE 6-3 KEEP A LOG

BUY a little notebook and keep a crystal log. When you are sober and motivated, draw seven columns on each page and label each column with the following:

Date (When you used crystal)

How (How you used crystal—snorted, smoked, slammed, booty bumped, etc.)

Amount (How much crystal you used)

Cost (How much you spent on crystal on that day)

High Rating (How good was the high on a scale of 0 to 10?)

Notable Events (Did anything notable happen? Did you finally approach the attractive person you've been too shy to meet? Did you finally finish your work project? Did you catch an STD or unintentionally become pregnant?)

Crash Rating (How intense was the crash on a scale of 0 to 10?)

TABLE 6-1

Sample Log

Date	How	Amount	Cost	High Rating	Notable Event	Crash Rating
8/2/2004	Snorted	1/2 g	$75	7	Amazing sex	4
8/9/2004	Smoked	1 g	$125	9	Amazing sex	–
8/10/2004	Smoked	1 g	0—had sex w/dealer	7	Amazing sex, blood from anus	8

Keep it simple so that if you are using crystal or you are recovering from a crash, filling in the information will require minimal effort. It should take you one to two minutes maximum for each entry.

Periodically review your log. Over time, was there any change in the frequency or amount that you used crystal? Even you don't see any change, keeping a log, or even a more detailed journal, will help you see more clearly what role crystal plays in your life and if that role is changing over time. Instead of turning a blind eye to your drug use, you will be more aware of your usage pattern and any consequences of using you may have—both good and bad. This will help you to keep your use in check, and alert you if you are starting to lose control.

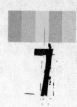

7

TAKING A LOOK AT CRYSTAL IN YOUR LIFE:
Is Tina Just an Occasional Visitor or Has She Become the Houseguest Who Just Won't Leave?

THIS CHAPTER EXPLORES how crystal fits in your particular life and what role it plays for you. This understanding is important for any person who uses crystal, whether you are an occasional partier or a heavy user, a person in recovery who is trying to stay clean, or someone who wants to continue using crystal while staying safe and trying to keep it under control. Do you use it as a fun party drug? Is it a way to deal with feeling bored? Does it help combat feelings of shyness? Is it a way to help you feel better about yourself? Is Tina the houseguest that was so fun and exciting when she first arrived, but now she is torturing you because you cannot get her out of your life?

WHAT ARE YOUR OWN REASONS FOR DOING CRYSTAL?

IF YOU USE crystal, there must be something good about it. Unless someone tied you down and spooned it into your nose, you chose to try it. If you did it again after the first time, there must have been something positive about the first experience that made you go back for more. What was that reason for you? Did new reasons develop over time? After hearing so much talk about crystal as a demon, let's look at how at times it may have seemed like an angel, helping you feel better in some way.

Studies find that social or cultural groups in different parts of the country have distinct usage patterns, though even within those groups, each individual uses crystal for his or her own reasons

Gay men commonly report using crystal at circuit parties and discos and in sexual contexts, such as sex parties/clubs, Internet hookups, or other sexual encounters, as well as during nonsexual activities. Among gay men, some who have HIV also use crystal to avoid depressive thoughts, loneliness, and concerns about physical attractiveness thought to be lost because of their illness. In addition, the power and confidence that crystal gives them is a strong antidote for the powerlessness many of them feel about HIV.

Heterosexual men and women reported different motivations. A 2004 study by Semple, Patterson, and Grant at the University of California–San Diego found that primary motivations in this group were "to get high, to get more energy, and to party," as opposed to enhancing sexual experiences. Nonetheless, this group was still found to have significantly increased sexual activity, with an average of 9.4 sexual partners in two months, with an average of 21.5 unprotected vaginal sex acts, and 41.7 unprotected oral sex acts during that time. A recent study by the California Department of Health was the first to find that sexual activity among heterosexual men appears similar to that of gay men, taking more risks: increased number of female partners, more frequent anal sex with women, higher likelihood of having sex with an injection drug user, and higher likelihood of having exchanged sex for drugs. Clearly, even for heterosexual people, meth has a powerful sexual effect.

Work is another common reason some people use meth. Manual laborers working several jobs, as well as wealthier urban professionals in high-pressure jobs with long hours, use meth to increase their productivity and their ability to work longer hours.

In contrast, many people in the rural areas report using meth to combat the boredom of living in quiet communities with little to do. It can help even the most empty life feel vibrant and exciting.

Some, especially young females, seek meth's ability to decrease appetite and cause weight loss. Severe obesity is still one reason that some doctors in other parts of the world legitimately prescribe pharmaceutically produced methamphetamine. Many people with eating disorders, such as anorexia, and body image problems turn to meth as a diet aid. The clinical picture then becomes even more complicated: anorectics typically see as overweight and unattractive, no matter how skinny and malnourished they become, and they need to keep starving themselves to get even thinner; however, meth boosts self-esteem and self-image, blinding addicts to the grisly reflection they see worsening in the mirror. Anorectics hooked on meth have a particularly complex self-image that fuels both their eating disorder and their drug use. The reflection is a combination of good and bad, ultimately reinforcing their belief that using meth and losing weight is good for them.

HAVE THERE BEEN PROBLEMS IN YOUR LIFE BECAUSE OF CRYSTAL?

DEVELOPING AN ADDICTION to meth is a process that, in most cases, occurs gradually. If you are still early in your drug experience, or if you use only once or twice a year, you may not have had any problems with addiction. At least not yet.

If you use crystal a little more frequently but are not at the level of partying every weekend or using every day, then be careful—watch for any potential problems that may be lurking so that you can catch them as they develop. You are in the blurry "intermediate zone," in which you actually may not have problems with meth, or if you do, they are not obvious or dramatic. They may seem so trivial that few people, including yourself, would consider them alarming. This intermediate zone is a tricky place to be because you may be teetering on the edge of addiction but there are no big red flags to warn you of the danger. If you are in this stage, actively assess your situation and how much control you really have. Your life may seem fine now, but a downward spiral could be just around the corner.

If you are a hardcore user, using most days or using regularly with out-of-control binges, and you have already experienced significant problems, such as losing friends, becoming estranged from your family, losing your job, failing in school, stealing or prostituting yourself to support your habit, or jeopardizing your health and catching an illness, such as HIV, *you are an addict*. You may realize this and sincerely want to stop. Many people, however, even in the face of serious problems, are still in denial. They tell themselves countless excuses and rationalizations to convince themselves that nothing is wrong: "Those people really weren't my friends anyway. Now that they don't call, I have more time to enjoy myself and use crystal." "My family never really understood me anyway, who needs them?" "HIV isn't so bad—it's a controllable disease that can be treated, so I don't have to worry. What's the big deal?" Or "I was planning on quitting that job anyway. I'm glad that I'm finally out of there."

Have there been negative consequences due to your crystal use? Are you being honest with yourself about what they are or how much crystal has changed your life? Are you honest with yourself about how important those changes are to you, or have you been coming up with rationalizations similar to the ones above?

THE DECISION MATRIX

A USEFUL TOOL to help you understand how crystal affects your life is the Decision Matrix, a tool to screen for alcoholism that was developed by an addiction psychologist named G. Alan Marlatt. It is called a matrix because it is a grid, looking at both the positive and negative ways in which crystal affects you. An example of the matrix is shown in table 7-1, and a sample matrix with one person's responses is shown in table 7-2:

TABLE 7-1

Decision Matrix		
	Positive, Helpful	**Negative, Problematic**
USING CRYSTAL: Immediate Consequences		
USING CRYSTAL: Delayed Consequences		
STOPPING CRYSTAL: Immediate Consequences		
STOPPING CRYSTAL: Delayed Consequences		

TABLE 7-2

Example of a Decision Matrix		
	Positive, Helpful	**Negative, Problematic**
USING CRYSTAL: Immediate Consequences	I feel high. I feel confident. I feel sexy and attractive. I've finally been able to lose weight and keep it off. Sex is intense and amazing. Sex is not as painful and I can go for hours. I do amazing things in sex I never would have dared before. I have great energy. I accomplish lots (at home, school, or work). I feel quicker and smarter. I enjoy music and dancing more. I can meet sexual partners more easily.	I can get anxious, jittery, or panicky. Sometimes I get chest pains. I can feel paranoid about other people. I can become aggressive and have gotten into fights. I have had hallucinations of voices. I don't bother with safer-sex precautions. I'll keep having sex, even if I notice I'm bleeding and should stop. I've contracted sexually transmitted diseases. I gave someone else HIV. I got someone pregnant unintentionally.

	Positive, Helpful	Negative, Problematic
USING CRYSTAL: **Immediate Consequences** (*Continued*)	I can meet sexual partners more easily. I feel more interested in things even when there's not much to do at home.	I forget to take my HIV medication because I'm so focused on sex when I'm high. I get into arguments with my partner or family. I spend hours on the Internet, like I'm stuck. I putter around at home & do things that later seem stupid, like taking apart my stereo. I've lost interest in food. I spend huge amounts of money on crystal, even when I haven't paid my rent or other bills.
USING CRYSTAL: **Delayed Consequences**	I feel more a part of my group of friends. I feel more a part of the glamorous crowd at circuit parties. I do better during exam crunches and pull up my low grades. I don't have to deal with relationship problems because I just have good sex. I have a big group of friends who share my interest in crystal.	I have a terrible crash. When I'm not high I feel depressed, tired, and unmotivated. I've felt suicidal during a crash. I miss work because I can't stop partying. I've missed work because I felt so terrible during the crash. I lost my job. I care less about my family and friends than I used to. I have lost weight I really didn't want to lose. I got HIV. My HIV or general medical condition are worse. I've begun stealing or prostituting myself to pay for more crystal.
STOPPING CRYSTAL: **Immediate Consequences**	No more crashes. I don't put myself at risk for STDs. I feel more emotionally intimate with my partner—with the pressure off, we can make love better.	I can't hang out with my usual social group. I miss the high. I don't feel as confident. Sex is not as intense or satisfying.

	Positive, Helpful	Negative, Problematic
STOPPING CRYSTAL: **Immediate Consequences** (*Continued*)	My mood is a lot more even and stable. I can pay my rent this month. My appetite has returned.	I can't suddenly fix bad feelings. I'm bored out of my mind. I can't work or study as hard or as long as I used to. I'm gaining weight again. I feel unattractive.
STOPPING CRYSTAL: **Delayed Consequences**	My health is improved. I have more energy in general. I've regained or improved my relationships with my partner, family, and friends. I spend less money, paid my debts, and even started saving money. I don't find myself in the same dangerous situations or with dangerous people. My general work performance and attendance have improved. I'm able to achieve important things in my life like getting a promotion or saving money for investments or retirement.	I'm losing my core group of social friends. I can't enjoy circuit parties or clubs anymore. I can't seem to keep my friends if I don't do crystal with them. Now I have to deal with my HIV and can't just live in the moment enjoying myself. Now I have to deal with difficult situations and feelings, and I can't just make them instantly disappear. Without my core group of partying friends, I feel alone and isolated.

To give you space to write in your answers, each quadrant is written on a separate worksheet. (See Decision Matrix Questions 1 through 4, pages 71–77.) Under each question, there are 20 blanks to fill in. Try to come up with at least 20 answers for each question. Usually people can easily think of 4 or 5 answers. The reason to strive for 20 is to force yourself to think of all the small and subtle ways in which crystal affects your life.

QUESTION 1   WHAT ARE THE *POSITIVE* THINGS
ABOUT *USING* CRYSTAL?

STARTING an addiction exercise with this question surprises many people who are accustomed to hearing that drugs are so evil that nothing
can be good about them. From experience, however, you know that this
is not true. If there were nothing good about crystal, you would never
have tried it and continued to use it after the first time. When answering this question, think about how crystal makes you feel, what areas in
your life it helps you with, what good changes happen when you use it.
In addition to "It feels great!" try to be more specific. *How* does it make
you feel great? Does it give you more confidence? Does it make sex more
enjoyable? Does it break you out of your shell in social occasions? Does it
alleviate boredom or work or home? Some people say that using crystal
was the first time they felt happy in years. Think about your own personal reasons and how meth may have made you feel better.

QUESTION 2   WHAT ARE THE *NEGATIVE* THINGS
ABOUT *USING* CRYSTAL?

IF you have read the preceding chapters in this book, you already know
the harm crystal can inflict, and you've probably heard other people say
what terrible things it has done to them. However, if none of those things
ever happened to you, then likely they don't have much personal impact
on you. In fact, if your experiences are completely different, you may feel
even more convinced that you don't actually have an addiction—how can
you believe all the bad hype if none of the things people say match your
experience? While it is helpful to hear about the many problems that
others experience from meth, it is most important to carefully consider
any harm that crystal has caused in your *own* life.

When writing your answers to Question 2, consider all areas of your
life. How was your mood during or after using crystal? Did it ever make
you feel anxious, panicky, or depressed? Have you ever heard voices or

become irrationally paranoid? Think about your behavior during and after using. Did you ever do something that you later regretted when you were sober—having unprotected sex, spending all your money, getting angry and yelling at a friend? Consider the effect crystal has had on people in your life—how are your relationships with your friends, your family, or your romantic partner? Has it had any affect on your work—have you ever come to work late, not felt up to the job, or completely avoided work and called in sick? Did you ever lose a job or come close to it because of meth? Did you start taking it to help with schoolwork but doing schoolwork gradually seemed less and less important than doing meth? Did you ever have any medical problems related to using? Did you spend more money on crystal than you wanted to, perhaps putting yourself into debt? Did you ever have to sell things, steal, or trade sex for money or drugs because you were so desperate to get more? To what extremes have you gone to get more meth? In addition to these examples, try to think of every possible aspect of your life where craving, using, or crashing may have adversely affected you.

QUESTION 3 WHAT ARE THE *POSITIVE* THINGS ABOUT *STOPPING* CRYSTAL?

THIS question may seem similar to Question 2, but with a twist. One way to gain a deeper understanding of how something affects your life, imagine what life would be like without it. Even if you don't think you need to stop using crystal, hypothetically what positive changes could happen if you stopped using? If you have intense crashes, could quitting help you feel less depressed or irritable? If getting high or crashing has disrupted your job, school performance, or relationships, could they be recovered or improved? If you add up all the money you spend on crystal in one month, what other things could that money buy? How about the money you would spend on crystal in one year? If you haven't been eating so well or taking your medications as regularly as you should when you are high, how do you imagine your health would be if you stopped using?

QUESTION 4   WHAT ARE THE *NEGATIVE* THINGS
ABOUT *STOPPING* CRYSTAL?

DESPITE Nancy Reagan's well-intentioned tactic to fight drug addiction, "Just say no," the battle is not so easy. While you identified many potential benefits of stopping crystal in Question 3, there will also be unpleasant things about stopping, whether it's the crash, finally facing difficult problems that crystal made you blind to, or the sheer torture of trying to resist the cravings. Would you miss it? If yes, then why? Would you miss the excitement? Would you miss the self-confidence it gives you? What would sex be like without crystal? If your social circle is a network of other meth users, what would it be like if you stopped getting high with them, or even worse, if you had to stop seeing them altogether? If you use crystal to help you work, how would stopping affect your productivity? Would you be able to keep up the fast pace that you'd set for yourself while using crystal? Would you be able to keep up with your boss's expectations after working as a meth-driven machine known for your extremely high level of productivity? Just saying no is not so easy because there are a lot of hurdles that will be difficult to jump over. If you don't examine the hurdles in an organized way and systematically figure out how to clear them, they may seem overwhelming and insurmountable. If that happens, you may just surrender and decide to keep using.

If you are having trouble coming up with 20 answers for each question in the Decision Matrix, use these general categories as guidelines:

- Specific mood before, during, and after using crystal
- General emotional well-being
- Physical health
- Money
- Time
- Relationships (family, friendships, romantic relationships)
- Job
- School
- Activities/boredom
- In general, how is your life different now compared to before you ever tried crystal?

DECISION MATRIX QUESTION 1

What Are the *Positive* Things about *Using* Crystal?

_____

_____

_____

_____

_____

_____

_____

_____

_____

_____

_____

_____

_____

_____

_____

_____

_____

_____

_____

_____

_____

_____

_____

_____

_____

_____

DECISION MATRIX QUESTION 2

What Are the *Negative* Things about *Using* Crystal?

_____

_____

_____

_____

_____

_____

_____

_____

_____

_____

_____

_____

_____

_____

_____

_____

_____

_____

_____

_____

_____

_____

_____

_____

_____

DECISION MATRIX QUESTION 3

What Are the *Positive* Things about *Stopping* Crystal?

_____

_____

_____

_____

_____

_____

_____

_____

_____

_____

_____

_____

_____

_____

_____

_____

_____

_____

_____

_____

_____

_____

_____

_____

DECISION MATRIX QUESTION 4

What Are the *Negative* Things about *Stopping* Crystal?

REVIEWING YOUR ANSWERS

How DID THE experience of filling in these questionnaires feel? What do your answers tell you? Were you surprised by how many ways meth actually helps you? Was it difficult to think of 20 negative consequences of using? After a little practice, did you start to identify the negative consequences more easily? Did you realize how many different parts of your life crystal affects? If you use crystal more than just a couple of times a year, then likely it's had some effect on many, if not most, of the general categories listed in the suggested guidelines for this exercise.

This section provides some ways to use the information from the Decision Matrix to explore your relationship to crystal even further. It may also give you a better general understanding of yourself as a person, aside from aside from drugs—e.g., what difficult areas in your life does crystal help you with, and if you stopped using drugs, how would you cope with those problems? If you want to stop using, this section will show you how to use your answers from the Decision Matrix to assist you along your road to recovery.

Question 1: What Are the Positive Things about Using Crystal?

If you are unsure if you have a problem with crystal, starting with your positive experiences with may feel like a safer place to begin self-exploration. This book does not write off crystal as something completely evil. Rather, it emphasizes the importance of understanding the drug from all sides to protect yourself from the extremely high risk of addiction. How significant are your positive experiences? If positives outweigh the negatives, you may decide not to stop using crystal—at least not now. If the positives don't seem worth the problems that crystal causes, then you may decide to stop using crystal. Get all the information you can about the drug and yourself, including the pleasures of crystal, so that you can try to make a rational assessment of the drug's place in your life.

Even if you know that you need to stop using meth, identifying and acknowledging your positive experiences on crystal is important. Sometimes when people are so strongly determined to stop using, they actually block out the good memories, saying with firm conviction that there was never anything good about a drug that caused them so much harm. This is called the "honeymoon period," when people feel so determined to be sober that they build up a false security and feeling of invincibility over crystal that leaves them unprepared when cravings return. You can't work successfully toward recovery without a complete understanding of your drug experiences. If you hide information about your drug use, whether good or bad, then your recovery is doomed.

In addition, recalling the good, as well as the bad, is an essential part of saying goodbye to a drug, which can feel like an old and intimate friend with whom your relationship has turned destructive. Saying goodbye is a long process similar to mourning, in which you reflect upon your memories and experiences, struggle with the idea of living without your old friend, and eventually learn how to move on with your life. If you don't acknowledge the good memories, you never go through the emotional challenge of letting them go, and the happy memories stay hidden inside you, holding on strongly to the hope that you will use again. With time, those lingering positive memories grow into idealized fantasies that downplay the uglier consequences of drug use. This distorted idealization is called "euphoric recall," which can seductively lure you back into using.

Most important, identifying the ways that meth has been helpful to you may clarify significant problems in your life that need work. Perhaps crystal masked low self-esteem or provided a temporary Band-Aid for underlying depression. Maybe using meth was the only way you could function at a job that made unreasonable demands on you. Once you clearly see the problems that crystal hid, you have an opportunity to actually fix them and make a profound improvement in your life.

On the other hand, if you don't address the fundamental problems that crystal covered up, those difficulties will never get better, and the urge to reach for drugs will keep coming back. If you realize that you use crystal to help you with self-esteem, depression, or an eating disorder, the drug only hides the problem temporarily, and in the long run it makes it worse. These are all good reasons to seek the help of a mental health professional, such as a therapist or psychiatrist, so that these deep psychological issues can be solved in a healthy and lasting way.

If crystal helps you combat boredom, *why* is your life so boring? What can you do to improve it? Instead of chemically hiding the emptiness, be proactive and search for more interesting activities that meet your life goals—take a class in something you've always wanted to learn about, pick up a new sport, volunteer and learn more about the people and the world around you—whatever sparks a little interest, go for it. Address the *cause* of your boredom.

If this exercise has identified significant problems in your life, it is important to tackle the fundamental problem than to rely on temporary solutions that treat the surface only cosmetically. If you have a headache because of a brain tumor, taking a painkiller may knock out the headache, but the tumor is still there, and when the painkiller wears off, you feel bad again, if not worse. Left untreated, the brain tumor will eventually kill you, so hiding the symptoms is actually harmful. Now the importance of Question 1 becomes even clearer. Take t list and use it to identify areas in your life that you can improve. By addressing them with healthier and more effective means, you can improve your general quality of life, as well as keep yourself from slipping back into using meth.

Question 2: What Are the Negative Things about Using Crystal?

Now is the time to come clean and be as honest as possible with yourself about any problems crystal has caused in your life. Write down the worst things that you can remember, but also include the seemingly little things—while each one may only seem like an annoyances, if you find yourself writing a long list of them, you should begin to wonder why you use something that causes you so many problems. If you have trouble answering this question, go over it with a friend who knows you well and has seen you sober, high, and coming off crystal. It would be unusual if you couldn't think of a *single* negative consequence from using meth. In that case, you may have already developed a blind spot about your meth use, and that blindness will prevent you from seeing any problems with addiction growing worse. However, if even the help of your friend, neither of you can come up with any significant answers, then your crystal use may not be a problem at this time.

If you believe that you need to stop using crystal, this list of negative consequences is a wonderfully motivating tool to help you quit. Whenever you feel the urge to use meth, take out this list to remind yourself how bad things got when you used.

Choose the three *worst* consequences on this list and flesh them out.

For each, write a narrative describing that particular problem or specific incident in detail. For example, if you experienced a crash that made you depressed and suicidal, describe the experience in graphic detail, as if you were writing a movie script—include where you were, what you were doing, how you felt, what kinds of thoughts were running through your mind, and how painful the experience was. This is a technique called "playing the tape." When people crave crystal, their memory is often selective, and they have euphoric recall, remembering the enjoyable parts of their experiences. Even if they *rationally* understand the bad consequences, that knowledge has little *emotional* impact on them—it is overshadowed by the intense feelings of anticipating getting high again. By playing the tape, you force yourself to recall the bad aspects of meth, with as much personal and emotional meaning as you can make yourself remember. The memories need to be vivid and powerful to balance out the effect of euphoric recall. In addiction, the brain-reward circuit, which lies deep in the primitive brain, compels you to use again, sending signals to the logical cortex and tricking you to rationalize why you should use meth again. To counter this, you need more than logical reasoning—try to activate other deep brain structures, such as the amygdala, where emotional memories are stored, to *more fully* recall the painful consequences of using meth. Unfortunately, the amygdala is not as deep, primitive, or powerful as the brain-reward circuit, so it is still a tough battle. However, it's a battle that you can win.

Question 3: What Are the *Positive* Things about Stopping Crystal?

What improvements can you imagine in your life if you stopped using crystal? Would you have more money to buy other things? Would your personal relationships be any better? Would you function better at home, work, or school? Would your health improve? How do the benefits of stopping look next to the benefits of using?

If you are motivated to stop crystal, your answers to Question 3 can also be a great motivating tool. Devastation and loss are often the strongest motivators to stop drugs. But it is also important to have positive motivations. Together with the positive feelings that addicts associate with using meth, there are also moments of clarity that many have, when they see how far they've fallen, and they feel a hopelessness that they will never be able to be the successful and functional people they once were. Then the sadness of this realization becomes another reason to get high again. Giving yourself positive goals will remind you that you don't have to be an addict and that your life can be better. They can give you optimism that will pull you out of hopelessness that would otherwise keep you trapped in a cycle of using even more crystal.. Quitting is not just about avoiding tragedy. It is also about recovering lost people and opportunities, getting your life back, moving forward, and achieving even greater things in life. When trying to stay sober is a struggle that makes you feel that life is empty without crystal, use this list to remind yourself of the wonderful things that can happen if you quit,

Question 4: What Are the Negative Things about Stopping Crystal?

Are there any negative aspects to stopping crystal? If not, then you should quit. Considering the risk of developing a powerfully destructive addiction, if stopping were to cause no problems, why not stop before you develop an addiction?.

However, if you cannot think of *any* difficulties with stopping crystal but you use fairly regularly, you may be one of those people who says, "I can stop anytime I want to, I just don't want to right now." See exercise 6-1 in chapter 6 to see if you are one of these people.

Even for people who are not addicted, there are usually some negatives associated with stopping crystal, such as not being able to bond with those couple of friends who still use, or not feeling comfortable in some of the places you go to socialize.

If you are a severe crystal addict, your answers to this question could pose serious obstacles. For example, if your whole network of friends are meth users, then trying to get away from them could leave you feeling lonely and completely isolated. If using meth is now a requirement to enjoy sex, then how can you imagine ever having sex after quitting? If never addressed, obstacles such as these could frighten most people right back into using.

Question 3 may seem as if it were meant to discourage you from stopping crystal, but it is another important tool to help you manage your recovery. In the past, doctors were afraid to ask their depressed patients if they felt suicidal. They thought that asking about suicide might *introduce* the idea and *create* suicidal thoughts. Could they cause their patients to attempt suicide by mentioning it? Fortunately, psychiatrists found this was not true. If a person does not want to kill himself, then uttering the word "suicide" will not magically make him want to die. But if the doctor asks, and the patient admits that indeed he has been feeling suicidal, then both the patient and the doctor are now prepared to address the problem and keep the patient safe. Similarly, mentioning the difficulties of stopping crystal will not prevent you from quitting. If you try to stop using, then you will face the same difficulties whether or not you've written them down. However, if you forecast the difficulties that lie ahead and carefully prepare yourself, then you will be much better equipped to deal with the obstacles when they happen. If instead, you are completely unprepared and a difficult situation catches you off guard, it is hard to think on your feet because your addicted primitive brain is overwhelming you with signals telling you to use meth again; However, if you are prepared for the situation, you can kick into autopilot, and even if it feels as if you are reading lines from a script, you may be able to navigate your way out of a potential relapse.

For example, if you predict that you will feel terribly bored if you stop using, you should structure your schedule ahead of time to make sure you are busy. Arrange your day with a balance of work or classes, exercise, relaxation, and "working the program," meaning going to twelve-step meetings or recovery groups. Keep yourself occupied and interested, but not overloaded. Boredom and having nothing to do are common reasons that people relapse especially early in recovery.

If you know that disappointment in sober sex will make you long for crystal, you may have to take a break from sex entirely for a little while. When you are further along in your sobriety, you can work on relearning how to have sober sex.

If you know that you will feel lonely without your network of meth buddies, then this would be a good time to reach out to family and sober friends and try to rekindle old relationships that were casualties from your drug addiction. Alternatively, it may be time to start cultivating new friendships, ones that are based on something more meaningful to you than a drug. Community activities and sports that you enjoy are good places where you can meet new people with similar interests. Volunteering for a cause important to you will give your life new purpose and meaning, and you can meet new people who share your passion. If you can't find activities such as these in your community, twelve-step meetings, at CMA or AA, are excellent places to meet people who you know share the same goal as you of getting sober. They personally understand the struggles you are going through, so from the outset, you know that you share some important things with these people. Be creative and look around your community for different opportunities to meet new people who have something in common with you and who don't do drugs.

IF YOU HAVE put sincere effort into completing the exercises as honestly as you can, you should have a good idea of how crystal affects your life. Hopefully this will clarify whether you must stop using crystal or if you feel that you can continue to use with caution. If you are still unsure, go back to chapter 6 and read it again with the information that you gained from the Matrix Model, then see how things stack up.

HOW CAN YOU HANDLE CRYSTAL IN YOUR LIFE?

STRATEGY:
Learn the Basic Techniques for Stopping Crystal

Objectives:
- If you are not ready to stop, learn ways to handle crystal safely while you monitor your use to see if you are able to keep control.
- If you are ready to stop, learn some basic strategies to break the cycle of use.

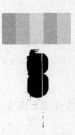

WHAT IF YOU USE CRYSTAL
AND YOU DON'T WANT TO STOP?

THIS BOOK IS written for people at any level of crystal use, from the person who has never tried it but is thinking about using to the hardcore addict who uses every single day. This chapter is specifically for those who have no desire to stop using crystal—knowing that it is a drug with a dangerous potential, they want to learn more about it to minimize any possible harm.

Let me reemphasize that methamphetamine is extremely addictive: the longer you use it, the more likely you will become an addict. Ideally, you should avoid it completely. Nonetheless, the truth is that not everyone is ready or willing to stop, and many of those who continue to use still care about their health and want to take precautions on their own terms—perhaps this is why you picked up this book.

This chapter is written for those of you in this group, recognizing that not wanting to stop crystal in no way makes you "evil" or "bad." You may be sincerely committed to being as healthy as you can, but you need to do it your own way, which may include not stopping drugs right now. If you are going to use, here are some suggestions on how to keep yourself as safe as possible.

In this chapter, you will learn specific strategies designed for the continuing user to monitor his or her meth use and to minimize any harm that might result from the drug. This approach is called "harm reduction."

WHAT IS HARM REDUCTION?

HARM REDUCTION IS a drug-treatment philosophy that emphasizes the importance of each individual's right to choose how to live. The guiding principle is to identify each person's self-determined goals—not only regarding drug use, but also a person's general life goals, such as relationships, friendships, career, and finances. The form of harm reduction treatment can vary, tailoring itself to help each person achieve what he or she wants. Focusing on people's personal goals helps to keep them motivated in the treatment—it is really their personal quest for health, as they define it. In this treatment model, a crystal user may strive for limiting crystal use to rare, occasional partying, more frequent but regular and controlled use, or even complete abstinence. All of these are considered acceptable treatment goals, as long as the motivation is to keep oneself as healthy as possible.

If you had questions and concerns about your crystal use but you weren't sure you had a problem, and you didn't want to stop partying, where would you go? What if all meth programs welcomed only people who promised to stop crystal immediately? Understandably, many people are offended when abstinence-based programs are uninterested in their personal goals, which may not include quitting meth. Instead, they perceive a blanket condemnation of all crystal users, which feels insulting and deters them from ever turning to medical or addiction professionals in the future, even when they know they need help. Harm-reduction programs are an important resource for addicts; instead of alienating them from the medical system, it offers them help in whatever way they are ready to accept.

You may want to educate yourself about crystal so that you can figure out the safest way to party. If you're questioning the possibility that you have an addiction, you may want an unbiased person to examine with you how you've been using crystal to see if you are still managing it well or if it has started to get out of control. You may want to know if you have any medical or emotional problems due to your meth use, so you can decide for yourself if you need to stop using. And you should be able to get these services in a nonjudgmental setting that will not turn you away if you're not quite ready to stop yet. The decision to stop needs to be yours, not someone else's. Harm-reduction programs were established to meet these needs, to reach out and engage meth users who would otherwise turn their backs on the medical and addiction communities.

When there are no harm-reduction services, some people who don't really want to quit obtain the social and medical services they need by lying about their drug use or their intentions to stop. But lying can be dangerous because the treatment that they receive is based on false information. If the treatment involves medication, then this can be particularly hazardous because some medications can interact negatively with meth. For example, the medication bupropion (brand name Wellbutrin) may help with depression and cravings for crystal. However, taken together with crystal, it can cause seizures.

Lying also sets up a poor relationship between the meth user and the health-care provider because it lacks sincerity and trust. Ideally your health-care provider should be your confidant and advocate, someone who will not judge you but will try to give you the best advice.

Most continuing crystal users do not lie about their use. They simply don't bother to seek any care. Some are blind to their health problems because they are so caught up in meth use. However, many people who fully realize they are medically ill have lost trust in the medical establishment. Their wariness of the medical system may prevent them from getting necessary treatment, even when they know they are seriously ill. Harm-reduction programs try to prevent addicts from developing this attitude so that they are willing to get help when they eventually need it.

Are there harm-reduction programs in your area? Currently most major cities have some harm-reduction programs, which may vary from simple drop-in information centers to harm-reduction counseling facilities. If you do not live in one of these cities, contact an organization in a major city closest to you; the staff may be able to direct you to services in your area. Some may also be able to provide limited counseling over the telephone, such as answering basic questions about crystal or providing crisis management.

HOW CAN YOU USE CRYSTAL SAFELY?

CONTROLLING CRYSTAL CAN be tricky because you are using a drug that physiologically tries to hijack your brain and convince you to keep using it, as well as to continue other behaviors you may associate with it, such as sex, Internet hookups, or going out dancing. Before partying with crystal, prepare yourself ahead of time to maximize your ability to stay within the limits you set for yourself *when you are sober*. If you are completely honest with yourself, you know that you may not have complete control over yourself when you are high, so before you start partying, set up some *external* controls to keep things in check. A little planning can go a long way.

Decide How Much You Are Going to Use

- Wherever you do crystal—at home, at a friend's place, at a sex club, at a disco or circuit party—decide beforehand how much you plan to do and how long you intend to party. While you are sober, set a realistic and "healthy" limit, and make a decision to stick to it. When you are **tweaking** (high on crystal), your perception of how much is "healthy" will probably be much higher.

- If you have ever found that doing more than a certain amount of crystal made you feel anxious or paranoid, or if it's ever made you hallucinate and hear, see, or feel things that were not there, set your limit below this.

- When setting your limit, don't forget to consider what the crash will be like. Many people feel tired and blue after partying, but if using more than a certain amount of crystal has made you extremely depressed or even suicidal, set your limit *below* this.

- If possible, buy your crystal before you go out, so you already have the maximum amount you plan to use. When you leave home, don't take your wallet, ATM cards, or credit cards. Carry an ID for emergencies and enough cash to get you home in a cab. Better yet, if you are going with a friend who is not drinking or using drugs, he or she can drive you, and you can leave the cab fare behind. Keep some emergency money on you, but bring as little as possible to prevent the possibility of buying any more crystal.

- If you are using at home, set aside the cash to buy the amount you decided to use, and if possible, give your wallet, ATM card, credit cards (you get the picture) to someone you trust to hold on to them so that when you reach your limit, you won't be able to buy any more, even if you want to. This may seem extreme, but be honest with yourself: if you've ever done crystal, finished your supply, and felt an uncontrollable compulsion to get more, you understand that this is an important measure that may help you stop when your tweaked mind says it still wants to party.

■ If you are going out and will be with people you don't know, keep your emergency money in a safe place (under the insole of your shoe, in a hidden pocket, or elsewhere on your person).

Plan How Long You Will Party

■ Decide how long you plan to use crystal, and decide on a length of time that is "healthy" and avoids negative consequences.

■ If you are a marathon partyer, is there a point in time after which using meth changes from being fun and exciting to being anxiety-provoking or scary? Is there a point after which you start to hear voices? Set your time limit safely before this.

■ Usually, the longer people party, the harder they crash, and the more depressed they become. Has crashing ever made you unbearably depressed or suicidal? If you know this time point, set your limit accordingly and stop using before this.

■ If you need to get to work on Monday, factor in recovery time, and plan to stop early enough so that your crash does not spill over into your next workday. If your crash lasts for twenty-four hours, then make sure you finish partying early enough to give yourself *at least* twenty-four hours to recover.

■ If you have HIV, which requires extremely tight adherence to your medication schedule, plan on breaks to take your meds at the right time, and if possible, set an alarm to remind yourself. Make sure that your medications are safe to take with your crystal: most HIV meds are safe, though some, such as the protease inhibitor ritonovir (brand name Norvir), are not because they will elevate your blood level of meth to toxic amounts. There are case reports of people who died from extremely high blood levels of methamphetamine when used in combination with certain HIV medications. Check with your physician, or contact one of the resources listed in the appendix to see how safely your medications mix with crystal. Many people assume it is not safe to take *any meds* when they party. Some people know their meds are safe but are too consumed by the drug high to take them. For whatever reason, many people skip their meds completely when they use meth. However, even brief drug holidays can allow HIV to become resistant to the medication. If you find that whenever you are out using crystal you never take your HIV meds on time, plan to finish partying before your next scheduled dose of meds.

Observe These General Precautions While Using Crystal

When you are partying, you may become so engrossed in doing more crystal and other activities that you forget to take the precautions you would ordinarily to take good care of yourself. Here are some important reminders:

- If you are doing bumps or snorting lines, never share straws, rolled-up dollar bills, keys, or "bullets." Always use your own. Snorting crystal causes damage to the mucous membranes in the sinuses, and there can be microscopic bleeds. If this happens, small amounts of blood, tiny enough to be invisible, can cover these snorting tools. Sharing these snorting tools increases the risk of catching or transmitting HIV, hepatitis B and C, and other illnesses.
- If you slam, never share needles and syringes. If you must share, clean your needles and syringes with bleach and water before the next user's turn, drawing the mixture through the needle and into the syringe to make sure that the inside of the needle is fully sterilized. If using crystal makes you too impatient to take the time to clean works properly, go to a needle exchange program and make sure you have your own works.
- Pace yourself. Decide how often you are going to do another bump, smoke or shoot up. If you get the urge to do more, check your watch to make sure you are not going too fast.
- Take a break every hour to rest and hydrate. Crystal makes you feel so energized that you don't detect your body's usual signals telling you that you need rest or fluids. Drink liquids with sugar and electrolytes, such as fruit juices or Gatorade, that will give

you much-needed calories. In addition, they will replace electro-lytes, such as sodium, calcium, and potassium that you lose in your sweat. These are very important for your heart to keep work-ing properly. Since crystal gives your heart a big workout, make sure to provide the optimal conditions for it to work its best.

- Fluids are also important for oral health. Dry mouth sets up a comfortable environment for bacteria to grow, and cavities and infections can occur much more easily. "Meth mouth" results from long-term crystal use, characterized by softened, misshapen, decayed teeth and bleeding, infected gums. If you perform oral sex while high on crystal, any sores or bleeding gums increase your risk of getting sexually transmitted diseases, including HIV and hepatitis. (see Meth Mouth photo, page 34)
- If you grind you teeth or clench your jaw when you are high, a mouth guard isn't the sexiest thing to wear out to a party, so try chewing sugar-free gum. This may provide a little more protec-tive cushioning than grinding your teeth directly against each other. Try chewing a gum such as Biotene, which promotes saliva secretion and contains xylitol and other ingredients that have some antimicrobial properties that may help to fight HIV. If you find that gum just makes you chew ferociously, try sucking on a sugar-free candy to see if this moistens your mouth and keeps it busy enough to stop grinding.

Take These Precautions if You Have Sex on Crystal

The intensity of sex is exponentially higher when using meth. For some, this is one its most appealing draws. Studies looking at motivations of dif-ferent types of users have found that gay men in particular sought more intense sexual pleasure from crystal. In contrast, heterosexual men and women reported other factors as more appealing. More recently, however, studies have shown that heterosexual men and women experience pro-found intensity when they have sex on meth. While sex may feel amazing, it poses two significant problems: (1) the more you have sex on crystal, the less appealing sober sex becomes, and eventually you may not be able to have sex without the drug; and (2) on crystal, the drive to have sex becomes so strong that important safer-sex precautions feel unimportant and even bothersome. Keep the following in mind when planning your next crystal-sex adventure:

- Always remember to use latex condoms and lubricant.
- Bring plenty of condoms with you because you will likely need more than just one, and you should not assume that there will always be condoms where you will be going. If you can't afford them, go to a local Planned Parenthood or Lesbian Gay Bisexual Transgender Community Center, where they are likely given out for free.
- When having sex, especially if you are continuing for a long time, periodically check to make sure the condom has not come off or broken. If you are the person who is being penetrated, periodically reach around and feel with your own hands whether your partner's condom is still intact. Do not depend on blind faith that your partner is keeping tabs on the condom. Take active responsibility for your own safety.
- Use plenty of lube—enough so that things stay slippery. Mucous membranes in the vagina, and more so in the rectum, are delicate tissues, and it does not take much to make them tear, though crystal can mask much of the pain from injury. The friction of prolonged, marathon sex can easily cause these tissues to bleed, so keep those surfaces slippery with lube. Remember, there is no such thing as too much lube, so pour it on.
- Do not use lubricants or birth control gels and creams that contain **nonoxynol-9,** a chemical used to kill sperm and prevent pregnancy. In test tubes, it was found to kill HIV, but in humans, it caused irritation to mucous membranes that *increased* the risk of transmitting HIV. Nonoxynol-9 is added to certain condoms, lubricants, and vaginal gels and creams to help prevent pregnancy. However, to protect yourself from HIV and hepatitis B and C, avoid using any products with nonoxynol-9, especially when you do not know the health status of your sexual partner..
- Silicone-based lubricants are probably better than water-based lubricants with latex condoms because they do not contain water and never dry up, so they last longer than water-based lubricants.

- *Never* use oil-based lubricants, which can cause tears in condoms.
- Even if you are the one penetrating others, if you have sex with someone with HIV, hepatitis, or any other STD, the germs are now all over the condom, and the next person you penetrate will be exposed to all those dangerous organisms. No matter what your role is in sex, whether penetrating or receptive, change condoms with each partner.
- If you see any blood, stop. You may not feel any pain, but if there is any injury, your risk of getting a sexually transmitted disease is high. If you are HIV-positive or have hepatitis, then there is a very high chance you could give it to someone else. Whether you are the person penetrating or being penetrated, periodically check for blood.
- When having oral sex, keep drinking liquids because the dry mouth that meth causes makes your oral mucosa more susceptible to cuts and abrasions, which can be entryways for STDs such as HIV and hepatitis viruses. Meth mouth is already full of potential entryways to catch diseases. Ideally, use a condom when having oral sex. With more people educated about how to prevent HIV transmission, the medical community has seen more people who report getting HIV from oral sex, even if they always used condoms for vaginal and anal intercourse. If you are unwilling to have oral sex without a condom, (1) try to visually inspect your partner's genitals for cuts or sores; (2) never let a someone ejaculate into your mouth; and (3) periodically check your mouth in the mirror because the high from meth and your determination to have sex may make you oblivious to injuries that can happen after hours of oral sex.

Anticipate and Manage the Crash

People have tried all sorts of remedies to help manage a crash, from taking high doses of vitamins and antidepressants to taking herbal supplements and drinking special teas. While many of these remedies are based on some theoretical knowledge about meth, it is not possible to make definitive suggestions because no rigorous studies have been found yet that support any of these anticrash methods. For example, it had been theorized that vitamin C, a powerful antioxidant, would protect the brain from damage by free radicals released when taking Ecstasy. However, one animal study found that vitamin C actually *increased* brain damage. Other studies have been inconsistent. And how do these animal studies translate to humans? Nobody knows yet.

Natural remedies are just as much of an unknown as pharmaceutical treatments. Just because they are "natural," they are no less potent or potentially harmful. Natural remedies work because their ingredients are biologically active—meaning they cause biological changes, just like pharmaceutically produced medicines. While moderate amounts of iron and calcium in your diet are good for you, too much of them are toxic. Other natural elements, such as arsenic, lead, and mercury, are frankly dangerous and potentially deadly. Regarding herbs and plants, be wary. Recall that hemlock and countless varieties of mushrooms can be deadly. Even kava kava, an herb and root commonly sold in health food stores for anxiety, has been found to cause liver failure and death. Rather than look for a magic pill, try to use these commonsense ways to soothe yourself to manage your crash:

- Eat, especially carbohydrates, which will quickly replenish your supply of needed calories. Despite the trend to eat proteins and avoid carbs, if you are dehydrated after a long period of partying, a high-protein load can damage your kidneys.
- Drink plenty of fluids with electrolytes. If you are dehydrated, your blood pressure will be low, you may feel more tired, and your kidneys will not get enough blood flow to sustain them. That can lead to kidney damage or even kidney failure. If you have HIV, then your kidneys are already at increased risk of disease, so take precious care of them.
- As you approach the time limit you set for yourself, start spacing your meth doses further apart, or take smaller amounts. This may be extremely difficult for some of you because you won't get as high, which is what your body and mind will be begging for, but tapering off more gradually will make the crash less sudden and severe.
- Make sure you are somewhere comfortable when you are coming down—your own home or a friend's place may be the best choices.

Keep your surroundings calm and minimize your exposure to things that are anxiety-provoking or bothersome.

- If you are having trouble settling down, keep yourself in a dark, quiet place. Too much stimulation can keep your mind running and not allow you to slow down. However, if a quiet place makes you more aware of your restlessness, try watching TV and flipping channels with the volume low to occupy your mind with the television and your restlessness with the remote control, without overstimulating yourself. Eventually you will start to wind down.

- Try meditating by closing your eyes and visualizing pleasurable scenes. Prepare a list beforehand of happy people, places, and things. (Keep crystal-related people, places, and things *off* the list, or you may find yourself back out there trying to get high again!) Keep your mind focused on these things, which will help keep your thoughts from sinking into darker places.

- When tiredness finally sets in, let yourself relax, sleep, and rest as much as you can.

- Expect that you will feel mentally and physically tired and that your mood may be erratic, irritable, or low. This is a natural part of coming down, and unless you are suicidal or hallucinating, you don't need to medicate these feelings—they will pass. Don't let them become excuses for using more meth or other drugs.

- If you are having sad, anxious, or angry thoughts, ask yourself if this is you or the crash speaking. Remind yourself that when coming down from crystal, everything can potentially be tinged with a negative color. Remember that this will pass. Sometimes simply knowing this can decrease some of the distress and help you wait it out.

- Do not make any major life decisions while you are high or coming down from crystal. Getting into arguments, ending relationships with friends or partners, or deciding to quit a job or move out of your home during a crash would be a big mistake. If you are feeling upset about something or someone, tell yourself you will deal with the problem after the crash is over. If the problem is real, it will still be there when you are feeling better, and you will be in better shape to make careful decisions.

- If you are feeling extremely depressed and you have any suicidal feelings, bring yourself to an emergency room or call 911. You can also call a local suicide hotline, where someone may be able to talk you through your depression or help you get more appropriate assistance. Meanwhile, keep reminding yourself that this is a part of the crash and that suicidal feelings will pass, and it is crucial that you keep yourself safe until they do. In this situation, medication can be very helpful, and in an ER, you can get medication that is helpful but safe.

WHAT IF THESE TIPS DON'T WORK?

THESE SUGGESTIONS SHOULD help you keep your crystal experience as safe as possible. If you try them but you are unable to stick to the limits that you set for yourself, or you continue to put your health, relationships, or job at risk, then your meth use is out of your control. Speak with a harm-reduction counselor to get other suggestions, and discuss whether now is the time to think about stopping the drug, before it completely takes over your life.

How much control do you have over crystal, and how much control does it have over you? When you are sober and well over the effects of a crash, make a list of things that you want in your life. Consider all areas: your general emotional well-being, intimate relationships, your sex life, your family and friends, school, your career, and whatever else is important to you. List to what extent crystal has helped you in these areas, and how much it has hurt. Be as honest as you can. Meth may help with many things on your list, such as boosting your self-esteem, improving your mood, and helping you to lose weight. But there are also a number of ways it may hurt you.

Review your lists: Are the benefits a fair trade for the problems? How many negative effects are you willing to tolerate? How many occasions of missing work are acceptable to you? How bad a crash is tolerable? How much risk are you putting yourself at for HIV and hepatitis? After deciding what is acceptable to you, don't just think about them, *write them down*—because if you become addicted, the order of your priorities will change: the pleasure you get from using will climb the charts to number one, and you will forget which things in life were most important to the non-addicted you. At that point you will lose the ability to rationally discern whether you are addicted.

If you find that the balance of control has shifted, that crystal now has more of a grip on you than you have on it, then the surest way to regain power over your own life is to stop using—and that means completely. If you have reached this point, then read chapter 9 to learn about ways to stop.

9

STOPPING CRYSTAL—
When You Feel That You Have Lost
Control of Your Life and You Want It Back

IF YOU FEEL that you have lost control over
crystal, or if you haven't yet reached that
point but want to make sure you never get there, you need to stop using
completely. While this is *my* strongest recommendation to you, for you
to be truly successful at this, the final decision to stop must be yours
alone. Addiction is a powerful deep-brain phenomenon, and it will
require intense work from the nonaddicted parts of your brain to battle
and overcome the addiction. But if you are willing to make the effort,
then you can win.

Through studies on humans and animals, through what scientists have
learned about methamphetamine's physiological effects in the brain, and
through accounts of people using crystal, it is clear that this drug is powerfully addictive. One of crystal's primary biological functions in the brain is
to make the animal exposed to it (in this case, that would be you) continue
to seek more. Crystal meth is an insidiously clever parasite whose primary
goal is to get you to take even more of it.

A good comparison is HIV—an ingenious virus that hijacks a person's immune system, the same system that a person uses to *fight* infections. HIV uses the immune system to its own advantage, luring immune cells to engulf it in its usual attempts to destroy invaders. However, HIV hides inside immune cells and then takes control of them so they do all the work of making more HIV and spreading it throughout the body.

Meth works almost identically. It hijacks the user's brain and eventually takes control, using it to control the mind and body to keep taking more meth. Like HIV, meth lives and works in the part of your body that would normally fight problematic behaviors, so it has weakened its most dangerous opponent. Repeated use of meth causes neuroadaptations—changes in brain structure and chemistry—altering the user's brain function so that judgment and decision making become weaker. As in the relationship of immune cells and HIV, the brain becomes blind to the danger of ingesting the drug (e.g., by going into denial, rationalizing, or making excuses for why crystal is not so bad). Because the addict is less consciously aware of the problem, crystal can take control. The brain's craving for it eventually becomes compulsive and automatic, and the degree of its control over a person's mind can be shocking. A person's life may be falling apart, with loss of job or severe deterioration in health, but the altered brain still convinces the addict to just keep on doing more crystal and that everything is just fine.

This powerful and insidious mechanism of methamphetamine is the reason that the only way to regain control or ensure that you will not lose control is to prevent any exposure to crystal. Completely. Otherwise, with the changes it slowly causes in the brain, you will lose the ability to distinguish between your own desires and those of the drug. During the act of using meth, the compulsion to continue using is the most intense, so stopping completely all at once will give you a better chance of success than trying to decrease your use gradually. As an illustration, people commonly report that while using meth, even if they stop feeling pleasure and have severe anxiety and paranoia, they still have a compulsion to use more, feeling as if they have become automatons programmed with the single purpose of getting more of the drug.

To avoid the trap, the most effective way to quit is to stop *completely*.

DETOXING

> Note: There is currently no FDA-approved medication for the acute treatment of methamphetamine withdrawal or the long-term treatment of methamphetamine addiction. The medications discussed here are based on current medical theories, results of recent medical investigations, and experiences with patients who agreed to use these medications in this way. I do not recommend that these medications be used as described unless you discuss fully with a physician their risks and benefits to you.

Unlike with alcohol and opiates, there is no universally accepted protocol for detoxing. This is unfortunate, because one of the greatest obstacles to quitting meth is the fear of the impending crash. Physiologically, crystal withdrawal is not dangerous—it won't kill you, as could happen in alcohol withdrawal. You will not experience tremors, seizures, delirium tremens with hallucinations, or death. However, crystal withdrawal can be debilitating and emotionally painful, and if depression becomes severe enough to make you suicidal, then indeed, quitting meth can be deadly. A detoxification regimen would help a great number of people who are having difficulty stopping because it would ease the pain and make the process less frightening—one less excuse that the hijacked mind can use to keep an addicted person from quitting.

The common experience of chronic users during a crash is extreme fatigue and low mood. They have difficulty experiencing pleasure, can feel depressed, and may even have suicidal thoughts. Appetite is greater, and the need to sleep increases but it is irregular: often someone crashing will sleep during the daytime, then have trouble sleeping at night. If you have these problems, it can be extremely difficult to reestablish a healthy, structured lifestyle. The frustration alone can spark a strong urge to start using crystal again—for many people experiencing withdrawal, restarting meth seems like the quickest and easiest way to feel better.

While there is no universally accepted way of detoxifying crystal users, there are many different strategies that doctors can use to help ease you through the experience. A good detox regimen should cover three basic areas. It should:

1. Decrease the intensity of the distress from a crash
2. Correct dysfunction or replenish levels of neurotransmitters in the brain to ease possible depression, fatigue, and other functional deficits resulting from the depletion of dopamine by crystal
3. Regulate sleep so that you fall sleep when you should (at night) and stay awake when you should (during the day)

Ideally, a medication regimen with these components should be taken while working with a substance abuse counselor who can support you through the process and keep you motivated, While the medications ease the discomfort of stopping meth, it is still a difficult process. Once the detox is complete, continuing the motivation to stay clean is a much greater challenge, one which a counselor can help you meet.

MEDICATIONS TO EASE PSYCHOLOGICAL DISTRESS

ONE OF THE most frightening experiences of crystal withdrawal and a major deterrent to ending a crystal binge is the depression, which can take various forms, such as dark mood, sadness, hopelessness, panic, and anxiety. There are several medications that can provide quick and safe relief when distress is unbearable. Unfortunately, the majority of these medications, called **benzodiazepines**, are potentially addictive and abusable. Some commonly known medications in this class are lorazepam (Ativan), clonazepam (Klonopin), diazepam (Valium), or long-acting alprazolam (Xanax XR). The regular form of alprazolam should be avoided because it has a particularly high addiction potential. Many addicts are already familiar with these drugs, since they are often sold by dealers to help cut the edge when meth causes too much anxiety or insomnia. In a detox, they are prescribed in a very controlled manner to make sure they are used therapeutically, instead of becoming another drug to abuse.

There are also other medications that are calming but do not carry the potential for addiction. Clonidine (Catapres), most often used as a blood pressure medication, works by blocking the release of adrenaline signals from a nucleus in the brain that can cause anxiety and distress. Clonidine is so effective that it is used in heroin detoxification, which can be excruciating. It has also been used as a nonaddictive treatment for the hyperactive symptoms of attention-deficit/hyperactivity disorder.

Pregabalin (Lyrica) is a recently developed medication that blocks calcium channels, which affect nerve transmission. It is currently used as a medication for neuropathic pain (pain from nerve damage due to illnesses such as diabetes, herpes zoster, or HIV). Preliminary studies show that it can be as effective as robust doses of alprazolam and lorazepam in reducing anxiety. Though is it chemically related to GABA, it does not attach to GABA receptors or other receptors associated with addictive drugs. However, if it is used regularly for a prolonged time, there can be some withdrawal discomfort. Moreover, in two studies, a small number of people reported experiencing mild euphoria from pregabalin, so the drug may have some addictive potential. Nonetheless, preliminary data suggest that it is much less addictive than the benzodiazepines, and at least two early studies have shown it to be as effective as lorazepam and alprazolam for treating anxiety.

MEDICATIONS FOR REVIVING THE BRAIN'S NEUROTRANSMITTER SYSTEM

CRYSTAL CAUSES SUCH a powerful release of dopamine in the brain that the reserves are depleted and dopamine function in the brain is significantly impaired, and it may take several days to weeks to restore enough dopamine to improve mood, energy, memory, and clarity of thinking. Therefore, medications that increase dopamine levels theoretically may aid recovery. Medications such as bupropion and amantadine (Symmetrel) are nonaddictive and can safely increase dopamine levels without any risk of addiction. Early results from a study currently in progress show that bupropion (Wellbutrin) is helpful with meth recovery and may even protect some brain cells from the damage caused by meth use. Earlier fears that bupropion would increase the risk of seizure were not seen in recent studies, and some of the subjects reported less of a dramatic high from crystal, perhaps resulting in using less and shortening the length of binges.

Another dopamine-like medication is ropinirole (Requip), which targets dopamine receptors in a nonaddictive way. Unlike the other dopamine-related medications, which often boost energy, many people find ropinirole sedating. It may be helpful to take it in the evening when you want to sleep, and also during the daytime if you have anxiety. By stimulating dopamine receptors, it may satisfy brain cells that feel the lack of dopamine. This use of ropinirole in this manner is theoretical and has not been proven in any clinical studies at this time.

Stimulants, such as methylphenidate (Ritalin, Concerta, Focalin, Metadate), pemoline (Cylert), or amphetamines (Adderall, Dexedrine) should be avoided because their activity in the brain is similar to that of methamphetamine, though at a much lower intensity. Stimulating the same brain pathways can stir up some of the old feelings of crystal use and put you at serious risk of relapsing. One recent study found that methylphenidate decreased cravings for crystal in some subjects. However, it is not clear what this means in the long term. Will crystal addicts continue to stay clean and sober, or are there other risks that methylphenidate may cause? This is only the first study, and the validity and the interpretation of the results are not yet clear. Before meth addicts rush to their doctors asking for methylphenidate, here is a cautionary example to keep things in perspective: Several years ago studies showed that gamma-hydroxybutyrate (GHB), a popular club drug, was very effective in treating withdrawal and decreasing cravings in alcoholics. Taken at face value, this study implies that alcoholics should use GHB to stop drinking. Unfortunately, GHB has also been found to be a much more addictive and dangerous drug than alcohol, with many deaths related to its use.

The last medication I will discuss in this section is **modafinil** (Provigil). Modafinil has been getting much attention in the medical literature because of promising effects in early studies with cocaine addicts (who may be neurochemically similar to crystal addicts). This medication seems to increase cortical activity (activity on the surface of the brain), which is normally low in heavy crystal users. It also improves energy and attention, which is a benefit that many meth users miss during recovery, feeling flat and tired without the drug. It may also help balance brain function that would otherwise have led to cravings and relapse. However, modafinil does not have significant dopamine activity, so it is considered to have low addiction potential. While this seems like the perfect medicine to help crystal addicts, there have been a handful of case reports of people feeling some euphoria from modafinil, which reminded them of crystal, and they experienced heightened cravings. This occurred with one of my own patients, who started taking increasing doses of modafinil in an abusive way. Fortunately, he was extremely motivated to stay clean and he never relapsed to using crystal. Another patient who had a history of past drug use but was not a crystal user tried modafinil and experienced severe LSD-like visual hallucinations that were terrifying. The lesson is simple: be cautious with any drug; even the most promising remedies have some risk.

THE IMPORTANCE OF NORMALIZING SLEEP

A MEDICATION TO help you sleep may seem unnecessary because most people feel exhausted and sleepy when crashing from crystal. However, if you look carefully at your sleep pattern, you may find that while it is easy to doze off in the middle of the day, nighttime often brings frustrating insomnia and fitful sleep. Instead, strive to establish a sleep/wake schedule that is well structured and leaves you feeling well rested. Structure is crucial to recovery, and this includes the simple act of sleeping at night and waking up in the morning. Put yourself back on schedule with the rest of the world so that you stay out of the "drug addict" routine. This will help you get back on your feet so that you can begin to work on important things in life—your drug recovery program, going to work, and taking care of the day-to-day business of life.

Trazodone is a powerfully sedating, nonaddictive antidepressant, which in small doses can be an extremely effective sleep aid. Other sleep medications include antihistamines such as diphenhydramine (Benadryl), chlorpheniramine (Chlortrimeton), and hydroxazine (Atarax). Diphenhydramine and chlorpheniramine are found in common over-the-counter sleep aids, such as Sominex and Unisom. A recently developed medication called ramelteon (Rozerem) stimulates melatonin receptors M_1 and M_2, the receptors in the hypothalamus that tell your brain when it is time to sleep. It has a stronger effect than melatonin and is not addictive, but not all people find it beneficial.

Avoid "benzo-like" medications, such as Ambien, Sonata, and Lunesta, which target the same brain receptors as benzodiazepines, but in a slightly different way. They are excellent for getting people to sleep, but they are also easily abusable, causing psychotic symptoms, such as hallucinations, which some people will try to experience recreationally. In addition, when taken in doses larger than the manufacturer's standard recommendation, these medications have the same addictive potential as benzodiazepines. Usually experienced drug users either know about the recreational effects, or they quickly find out. Therefore, the principle of "if one works, two should be better" definitely does not apply with these medications.

In addition to hallucinations, benzo-like medications have been associated with a number of unusual activities that seem out of the user's control. This has been reported moreso for zolpidem (Ambien). For example, one woman woke up to find had she dismantled all her remote controls and neatly organized the parts on the kitchen counter. In another example, a man drove to his ex-girlfriend's home at four AM and banged on the door until the police came and shook him awake. These people were completely unaware of their actions, yet some of them ended up behind the wheel of a car, driving in traffic! These are not fun experiences because the people who have them can't remember them at all. However, they put themselves (and others) at risk of serious harm. If you are trying to clean up and stay sober, who knows where your unconscious mind could lead you in the middle of the night? These medications are even more dangerous because they are advertised as completely safe. They are not. Stay clear of them.

If you decide to try a detox regimen, you must do it under the supervision of a physician, ideally one with experience with addiction. When discussing possible regimens, be sure you tell your doctor *everything* that you take—recreational drugs, prescribed medications, over-the-counter drugs, herbal supplements, and even vitamins. The last thing you want when you are dealing with the challenge of quitting meth is an accidental drug interaction that could have serious medical consequences.

HOW TO USE A DETOX PROTOCOL: WORKING WITH A DOCTOR AND A TREATMENT CONTRACT

YOU MAY NEED one, two, or all three categories of medications to help ease the discomfort of stopping crystal. Most of these drugs require prescriptions from a physician, which may seem burdensome, but this is actually a good thing because it ensures that the process is being monitored by a health care professional. To detox, you *must* work with a physician. Ideally this should be in conjunction with a drug counselor, who can support you through the process of detoxing and coordinate other relapse-prevention services to make a comprehensive and effective program that is tailored to your specific needs.

Many experienced addicts know how to obtain the medications I've mentioned through drug dealers or by manipulating physicians, and the temptation to do this so that you can orchestrate your own detox will be strong. Instead, take yourself out of the drug-using world to accomplish this. Put an end to the drug-using mind-set of trying to control everything, and detox with the help of a physician. One of the hardest parts in this process may be giving up control to someone else who will decide what "drugs" you put in your body. Letting go of control is extremely hard, but admitting that you can't control everything is a fundamental principle that will help you out of your addiction. Ask yourself this question: If you really can control everything, then how did you get so addicted that you need to be detoxed? It is time to hand the reins over to someone else.

GUIDELINES FOR WORKING WITH YOUR DOCTOR

Your physician should set up a 10-day detox schedule for you after discussing which of the three categories of medications would be helpful for you and which specific medications would be safe. In order for your doctor to make these determinations, you must discuss *everything* that is possibly relevant—medical conditions you have, what drugs you've been using, and what medications you take.

Your doctor should give you prescriptions for enough medication to last only 5 days, which requires you to check in with your doctor at short intervals. Seeing your doctor frequently will keep up your motivation, put a little extra pressure on you to stay sober, and if you are having any problems, they can be addressed quickly. Meeting frequently will also reassure your physician that you have committed to getting off crystal and that this is not a scam for get drugs, something that many physicians are wary of and try hard to avoid. If your doctor sees that you are earnestly trying to get better and are disciplined enough to stick to this structured treatment, she will be much more open to trying a detox with you.

Day 6 is your second meeting with your doctor. That day, he should collect urine for a drug test. It is another assurance that you are trying your best and not just collecting scripts for meds to mix with other party drugs. It is best when the doctors have on-site testing, so you can see the results instantly and decide what to do if your urine tests positive. You both discuss whether it feels safe to keep trying or if you need to be referred to a drug treatment program that's better able to handle difficult addiction cases. In addition, knowing that you are going to have a urine drug test gives you even more incentive to try to stay clean. Shore up as many reasons as you can to be mindful and keep away from crystal.

If things are going smoothly with the detox, your physician should give you prescriptions to last you the remaining 5 days. Small prescriptions with no refills decreases the temptation to use more than your schedule directs. During a detox, you should see your doctor often. Picking up prescriptions for the rest of the detox is a good incentive to continue your contact so that someone is following your progress.

Your physician should draw up the following contract with you:

1. Your prescriptions are for 5-day supplies, no more and no less.
2. If you lose your medications, they fall down the sink, or you run out of medication for any other reason before 5 days, I will *not* provide you with any extras pills, prescriptions, or refills. The set amount you get is a one-time deal. These medications are important, so be careful and keep them safe.
3. Addiction is a chronic, relapsing, and remitting illness, meaning that as an addict, you may relapse in the future. However, if you require this kind of detox more than twice, this treatment is clearly not effective, and you would require more intensive treatment than this office can provide. In such a case, it would be clinically inappropriate for me to continue to treat you in a way that has proven to be ineffective, and I will *not* give you prescriptions for any more detox medications. *This in nonnegotiable.* Instead, I will help you find a drug treatment program where you will receive more intensive treatment for your addiction.

This contract is important for several reasons. First, your doctor needs to feel that he or she can trust you. Most physicians are uneasy about working with drug addiction, and many have been burned by patients lying to them in order to obtain controlled substances that they then abuse. Most doctors have had patients say they "lost their medications," or "accidentally dropped their meds down the sink," and they repeatedly ask for more prescriptions. While this happens frequently with controlled substances—medications that patients should be most careful with—for some reason, nonaddictive medications, such as laxatives and antibiotics, rarely get misplaced. Hence, most doctors are extremely wary of addicts seeking drugs. After such experiences, many doctors may not be willing even to consider trying a detox regimen. However, presenting your physician with this contract sets up parameters that can make your doctor feel confident that you are making an honest and sincere plea for help and that you are committing to work within a strict and safe plan that you both agree upon.

Setting a limit on the number of times that you can request this detox regimen prevents you from using it as regular way to end crystal binges, making you feel more comfortable bingeing more often. Even if you do not intend to keep bingeing, such a pattern can still develop. Making a contract with your doctor creates a safety mechanism, so that if detoxing and using your own resources to stop are not enough to quit meth, the contract automatically directs you to more intensive care, which you will likely need. Hardcore addicts will doctor-shop to get anticrash medications from several different physicians, but if you truly want to stop, (1) sticking with one doctor who knows you well, and (2) using the contract are the best ways to protect yourself and to help your doctor to feel comfortable enough to work with you. Show your doctor a copy of this chapter to fully explain the reasoning behind the treatment. If your request seems logical and medically sound, your doctor will be more likely to help you.

NOW THAT YOU HAVE STOPPED, HOW DO YOU STAY CLEAN?

Working on Keeping Crystal Out of Your Life

Objectives:

- Learn the concept of "relapse prevention"—not just a treatment but a way of living that will protect you over your lifetime.
- Learn what kind of "lifestyles" put you more at risk for relapsing.
- Identify situations, people, places and things in your life that may increase your chances of relapsing
- Learn lifestyle strategies that will improve your quality of life as well as reduce your risk of relapsing (e.g., how to say no, structure your time, reward yourself, and develop techniques to help you get through bouts of craving).
- Learn about the different kinds of addiction treatments. Understand what they really are (are the rumors true?), how they work, and what they offer, so that you can choose the best fit for yourself.

10

RELAPSE PREVENTION:
Working on Staying Clean

IF YOU HAVE decided to stop using crystal, you have successfully stopped, and you want to keep it out of your life, then likely you have gone through some deep soul-searching and difficult times to get this far. Congratulations! But now the really hard work begins. The single act of quitting was a monumental task, but it is only the beginning of a long road of maintaining sobriety. Determining how to stay off meth and lead a crystal-free life is a lifelong endeavor because addiction is not just psychological—it is also physiological, meaning that it is a physical process in the brain that occurs even if, intellectually and emotionally, you want to stay as far as possible from drugs. But do not despair—things become much easier with time.

The ambivalence and temptation to use crystal will always be a part of you, to some extent. Imagine two parts of you—one part wants to be drug free and healthy, while the other part wants to use meth again. Think of your mind as a corporation with two major shareholders competing with each other to get enough shares to control the company—in your case, this means making executive decisions about whether to use crystal. Relapse prevention tries to keep the clean-and-sober shareholder in control, not the addicted one who will eventually run the business into the ground. As aggressive competitors, both shareholders relentlessly vie for control. Therefore, you must be constantly vigilant for sneaky corporate takeovers by your addicted side.

Though addiction has many psychological symptoms, it is as much a medical illness as diabetes and high blood pressure. Looking at data on patients with high blood pressure, diabetes, and drug addiction—the statistics for how well people stick to treatment, how often they "relapse," or how often they have periods of worsening symptoms—it is difficult to discern any significant differences. All three are biological processes. The important take-home point is that like other chronic illnesses, addiction requires ongoing monitoring and care. Even after you achieve sobriety, you should not simply return to living life the way you had been before. Just as if you have been diagnosed with asthma, once you treat the acute illness, you need to make lifestyle changes to minimize the risk of another asthma attack. You must accept the fact that you need to treat and monitor your health for the rest of your life.

Understanding addiction as a chronic disease helps recovered addicts to keep aware of the constant threat of relapse in perspective, even after several years of sobriety. Even after twenty years of sobriety, the potential to fall back into full-blown out-of-control drug use is still there. The brain circuits of addiction may be quiet, but they are still there, and they can be activated and quickly return to a full relapse. There are countless stories of alcoholics and drug addicts who stayed sober for decades, but once they let their guard down and convinced themselves they were no longer addicts, they found themselves just as out of control with drugs as they had been decades before.

A helpful model is to think of addiction as an escalator that is constantly moving downward. You are standing in the middle of the addiction escalator, and if you don't move your feet, the rolling staircase will take you lower and lower, to the depths that addiction takes you. You have to walk or even run up the steps to rise to safety. Even when you are higher on the escalator, you must continue to climb just to stay in place and to prevent the escalator from bringing you down again.

In this model, climbing represents the work you put into recovery.

Given time, effort, and the length of your sobriety, the escalator will slow down, and it will feel less arduous to maintain your current level on the escalator. Eventually it will be even easier to climb and to move higher up in life, rather than just to stay in the same position. *But never forget that the escalator is always running.* If you convince yourself the escalator has stopped moving, you will stop climbing, meaning that you will forget about your awareness and your recovery skills. And the escalator will gradually bring you back down to the depths of your addiction.

The medical model emphasizes that much of the basis for addiction is biological. Studies of the brains of chronic drug users show substantial structural changes. Others studies, in humans and in animals, suggest that these brain structures are responsible for controlling addictive behavior—if they are damaged, the behavior is difficult to control. However, the difference between addiction and other medical illness, such as high blood pressure or asthma, is that the location of the malfunction is in the brain, so the illness affects feelings and behavior. For this reason, it is easy to understand why most people, including addicts themselves, see addiction as a personality issue, and they attribute it to bad choices made under free will, rather than to biological process. Society tends not to blame people for having high blood pressure or diabetes, and there is little shame in their seeking treatment for these illnesses. However, American culture views addiction as a weakness of character. It blames the person for being an addict, and the shame makes it even harder for the addict to admit to having the illness and to seek treatment.

By clarifying its medical nature, I hope to *destigmatize* addiction, making it easier for people to accept and treat. Under the medical model, a slip or relapse in drug use is similar to an asthma flare-up: the person with the illness is not "bad"; in a chronic illness, we expect that a slip is bound to happen at some time, though we work hard to minimize the possibility. Just like a patient with asthma, the addict should not focus on "being a failure" for relapsing—this is demoralizing, and delays treatment and recovery. Rather, a relapse or setback is an important time to investigate what caused the flare-up and how treatment needs to be adjusted or intensified to quickly get things back on track.

The medical model is not an excuse to let go and be apathetic about addiction. It is not a reason to shrug your shoulders and say, "Well, there's nothing I can do about it, it's inevitable, so I may as well keep using crystal." *Quite the opposite.* If a woman with diabetes found that her blood sugar was too high, it would sound unwise, if not ridiculous if she responded, "So what's the point of this insulin? I may as well forget about these meds and eat as much sugar as I want because I'll never get my sugar under control!" During a disease flare-up, whether the illness is diabetes or addiction, the affected person needs to tell his or her doctor what has happened, Together they can consider what changes in lifestyle and treatment are needed to get back on track.

WHAT IS "RELAPSE PREVENTION"?

RELAPSE PREVENTION IS an addiction treatment based on clinical principles for treating alcoholics developed by G. Alan Marlatt, Ph.D., one of the "founding fathers" of modern addiction treatment. The original model has been adapted to many uses, from chemical to behavioral addictions. The underlying idea behind relapse prevention looks at recovery as a continual learning process.

Older views of addiction were harsh and critical—sobriety was success, and if you relapsed, you were a failure. You were either sober or you were a hopeless addict. Without much room in between, many addicts felt that if they slipped back into drug use, they were hopeless failures, and addiction was their only lot in life. There was an unrealistic expectation that sobriety was as simple as understanding that there was a problem—the "epiphany" would magically take away the cravings and dangerous loss of control. Needless to say, this perspective on addiction was discouraging and demoralizing because the majority of addicts who try to stop eventually slip or relapse a number of times before reaching any significant length of successful sobriety. The older concept of addiction also made doctors and other health care professionals reluctant to work with addicts because addicts were almost all destined to be failures.

The modern concept of addiction does not consider a relapse to be a failure. In fact, relapsing is almost inevitable in the process of recovery. Many addicts use their frustration and feelings of hopeless failure as a rationalization or excuse to continue using drugs—why bother quitting if you will never succeed? Instead, falling down should motivate you to get up, dust yourself off, and try harder. Keep trying and eventually it gets easier—that's how babies eventually learn to walk. If babies gave up after their first few falls, we would all still be crawling.

BASIC PRINCIPLES OF RELAPSE PREVENTION

THE BASIC GOAL of relapse prevention is simple: to prevent relapse. The strategy is to identify the things in life that put you at risk and to figure out ways to avoid them. This is best done with the assistance of someone experienced, such as a counselor, a therapist, or a group, who can point things out that you may not see. The addicted part of your mind works insidiously and can distort your thinking and create blind spots, even when your conscious motivation to stay sober is strong. Ideally, you should avoid all things that pose a risk. However, in real life, it is not possible to avoid all risks. Therefore, relapse prevention also includes working on how to cope with risky situations effectively until you can get yourself to a safer situation. The basic schema is a chain of three related phenomena that can lead to drug use: situations, reactions, and coping skills, as illustrated in figure 10-1.

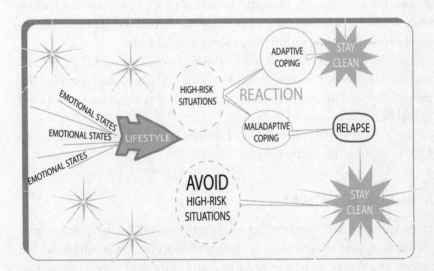

Figure 10-1 Relapse prevention theory.

The ways you live your life, or your emotional state, can bring you into a situation that is a high risk for relapsing. When you find yourself in those situations, how do you react? Right now your automatic reaction may be to use crystal, but there are other, better ways of coping that can get you through a high-risk situation without resorting drugs.

YOUR LIFESTYLE

How DO YOU live your life and what impact does that have on your emotions? Is your job too pressured and stressful? Are you unemployed or underemployed, feeling bored all day? Are you around people who use drugs, and do you feel pressure to do the same in order to feel part of the group? Are you unhappy or depressed and want to feel good again? Do you have low self-esteem but are trying to find ways to feel better about yourself? Do you have HIV and feel like a prisoner of it, wishing you could forget about HIV, even for a little while? Are you tense, irritable, and frustrated with your work, relationship, or family?

These are only a few of many important aspects of life that *all* people should think about. Problematic lifestyles that cause negative feelings often lead to relapse because addicts are accustomed to address negative emotions with crystal rather than change the lifestyle..

Take inventory of your lifestyle—the way you lead your daily life, the way you feel about yourself, and the way that you interact with other people. Are any of these things situations in which you have used meth to feel better?

See exercise 10-1, "Identifying Lifestyle or Emotional Issues," (page 130) to explore this further.

HIGH-RISK SITUATIONS

In ALCOHOLICS ANONYMOUS (AA), there is a well-known phrase, "people, places, and things." It is a reminder to think about which people, places, and things, as well as situations and emotional states, are risky for you so that you can steer clear of them. Having your crystal dealer's telephone number in your cell phone puts you at risk. The physical presence of your dealer, as well as friends and acquaintances who use, put you at risk. Simply seeing your dealer's number on your caller ID puts you at risk.

Places where you used to use crystal, such as your meth buddy's house, discos, sex clubs, and circuit parties may put you at risk. Access to the Internet in general may put you at risk.

Make a list of people, places, and things that are a high risk for you. This is your personal list of high risks to avoid. In particular, when you are newly sober and just beginning to develop better coping skills, you need to stay as far from these risks as possible. Give yourself a breather from those friends who use crystal. Stay away from clubs, sex parties, and circuit parties. Take a break from the Internet, where you may find yourself searching sex sites and then run off to a crystal-sex hookup. Throw out your dealer's telephone number and erase it from your speed dial. If your dealer sometimes calls you, tell him or her not to call you anymore, and if your dealer persists, change your telephone number. This may seem like a tremendous hassle, but the mere sound of your dealer's voice on the phone can bring back a powerful rush of feelings that may overwhelm your best intentions to quit. See exercise 10-2, "Identifying High-Risk Situations," (page 131) to explore this further.

There will likely be some items on your list of people, places, and things that are unavoidable. Your dealer may be someone in your neighborhood who passes you occasionally on the way to the store. You may need to use the Internet regularly for work. Consider which items on your list are unavoidable. If you are truly unable to get these things out of your life, then you need to plan how to cope with them.

Here are some examples:

■ If your computer is an essential part of your job and you depend on e-mail, the Internet can be a looming temptation. If you don't actually need the Internet for your job, uninstall the browser from your computer (you can always reinstall it if you discover that it is necessary). Getting rid of your Web access can block those brief compulsions to "just take a peek" at your old favorite sex sites, which could trigger old feelings and a strong desire to get high. If your job does require Internet access, have someone install a web filter (like "parental controls") on your computer that restricts any sex-related sites. You should not install it yourself because you can easily turn off the filter if your willpower is weak. Ask your company information technology staff to do this so that you don't accidentally damage the company network. Simply explain that someone has been using your computer to view adult sites, and you want to stop this from happening any further.

■ If you can't completely avoid people you used to do crystal with (friends, the local dealer, co-workers, your parents, your partner or spouse, etc.), think of the situations in which you'll see them and plan what you will say and do in each of them. If they start talking about the last time they were hanging out using crystal, the next big circuit party, or *anything* that may be a trigger, think of standard responses you can fall back on, such as: "Can we talk about something else?" Or politely change the topic to something that's not a trigger for you, such as: "Hey, how's your brother doing?" Practice the lines, even if they start to sound like a script. Eventually you'll get used to saying them, and if you always have the same response, eventually your friends will learn that you don't respond to conversations about their drug use or other drug-related topics. If a mouse keeps pushing a lever for food but nothing ever comes out, eventually the mouse will give up and stop pressing the lever.

■ If the people you can't avoid ask you directly to use crystal with them or invite you to a place where you know people will be using crystal, say "No thanks." Refusal skills are essential—you are firmly saying no to the people who are tempting you, but you are also firmly saying no to the addict part of you that always wants to take control. See the section called "Refusal Strategies" (page 121) for a detailed discussion of this topic.

■ If the people you can't avoid are people who live with you, such as a parent, a spouse, or a partner, and they refuse to stop using crystal, it's time to change living arrangements. One way or another, you need to keep your home a clean and safe place.

■ If you used to do crystal in your bedroom, what do you do? Every aspect of the room—the look, the smell, the place you sat when you smoked or the table you stood over when you snorted lines, will trigger memories and feelings that can powerfully pull you back to crystal. Short of moving to a new home, you will have to make some changes. Paint the walls a different color. Get different color bed sheets. Rearrange the furniture, and if possible, replace some things, such as the table you used to snort lines on. It's the same room, but when you sit in your chair from a different angle, and you see walls in a different-colored and with different pictures, your brain is less likely to feel the same cues it did when you were using crystal, and it will be less of a reminder of those times. Think of Pavlov's dog, which salivated every time he heard a bell because the sound of the bell was paired with receiving a steak. In this case, the bedroom is the bell, and meth is the steak that was paired with it. If you can't get rid of the bell, at least change the sound enough so it stops making you salivate.

There are many people, places, and things that can increase your risk of relapsing. However, as you can see, there are as many ways to deal with them if you aren't able to completely avoid them. The best strategy is to plan ahead so you can be prepared. Learn the danger zones you can avoid, and for the unavoidable, create a specific plan for how you will deal with each situation—even if you don't use that exact plan in the real situation, the planning process is empowering, and you are more psychologically prepared when you face the trigger. If you are caught totally off-guard in a high-risk situation, the urge to use may be so strong that you can't think well on your feet. Or more likely, the desire to use may become so strong that you will not *want* to think. If you are prepared, you won't have to think much because you'll already know what to do. You just need the inner strength to do it.

REFUSAL STRATEGIES

"JUST SAY NO." The catchphrase from Nancy Reagan's well-intentioned antidrug campaign sounds oversimplified, underestimating the power of addiction. However, combined with other strategies of relapse prevention, the ability to say no is extremely powerful. And difficult. This is why it is important to *practice* refusing. When someone suddenly offers you meth, there's very little time to think of what to say. Intellectually, you know you *should* say no, but will you be able to? If you have practiced the words, they will be easier to say. If you have practiced them until they've become *automatic*, they will be even easier to say, regardless of whether you sincerely mean them at the time. Early in recovery, you will be struggling against a powerful temptation to say yes. But that is irrelevant here. Your single goal is to get away from this powerful danger. *Just say no.* Avoid any interaction in which the powerful cue of meth that is being dangled in your face could possibly overpower any rational thought. You may continue to struggle against the wish to say yes, but without the crystal within reach, your logical side will have a better chance of staying in control.

Think of a common scenario in which someone offers you crystal, such as passing old drug pals on the street, or at the beginning of a hookup with someone you meet online. Think about how you want to come across to other people and what action would effectively end this dangerous situation. You want to feel and appear firm and unwavering, not indecisive and unsure. A dealer or other crystal users can sense ambivalence, and they know how to target your vulnerabilities. Don't be fooled by their generosity. Whether they are dealers or friends, they have selfish reasons to get you to use: The dealer obviously wants to make money. Even the generous freebie that gets tossed your way is just a ploy to get you hooked and back to being a regular paying customer. Other users want you to join in because it makes them feel less guilty about their own use—"Crystal can't be that bad if someone else is doing it, too, right?" Disregard whatever they tell you, and focus on your primary objective—to be clean and healthy. Tell them no. State it clearly and succinctly, without reservation.

Some possible ways to refuse are:

- "No, thanks, I'm taking a break from partying."
- "No. I realized that it's not good for me, and I'm trying to stop."
- "No. Crystal's become such a big problem everywhere you look, and I've decided I don't want anything to do with it anymore."
- "No. Crystal is really affecting my health, and I don't want to do it anymore."
- "No. I realized that I have a problem with crystal, and I decided that I'm going to stop."
- "No. I realized that I have a problem with crystal, and I decided that I'm going to stop. As my friends, I need your help with this, so please don't talk to me about crystal anymore."
- "No. I have a problem with crystal, and I decided that I'm going

to stop. I don't want you to sell it to me, and I don't even want you to talk to me about crystal again."

■ Or simply, "No, thanks."

Make eye contact when you say no, which shows sincerity and gives a nonverbal signal that you do not welcome a challenge to this statement. Never use expressions such as "I think" or "It seems like"; leave no room for possibility in your refusal. Keep the interaction brief. If you are in a situation where you have to talk to these people, change the subject completely and don't take the bait of being drawn back to it. Be a wall. They will keep trying to steer the conversation toward meth to undermine your determination. If they still do not respect your clearly stated refusal, it is clear how little regard they have for you. If you are surrounded by people who have no regard for you, if they are relentlessly pushing you toward danger, how does that picture look to you? Give yourself the respect you deserve and remove yourself from harm's way—leave.

Once you've written out your script, practice it with someone in a role-play. At first it may feel silly and you may joke about it. That is fine—enjoy yourself! Just remember that the reason you are doing it is serious—to save your life. Practice it over and over until it rolls off your tongue naturally and you hear yourself saying the words with natural confidence. In a real situation, you are not just saying these words to your dealer or your friend—you are also reminding yourself of your strong conviction. In a high-risk situation where your craving may be piqued, *hearing your own voice* state definitively that you will not use will remind you that the strong and healthy part of you is in control. Every time you say it, it emphasizes your determination to recover.

STRUCTURE YOUR TIME

WHEN YOU ARE first stopping crystal use, keep yourself busy. Put in writing a detailed schedule, not an amorphous list of possible activities you keep in your head, so that you have a committed activity or meeting with sober people scheduled for every hour of the entire day. This includes scheduling rest time, but with sober friends. Make a schedule for at least one whole week after quitting, and be especially careful to be safely occupied during the times you used to get high, such as on the weekends or after work. Make the activities a mixture of productive work and fun. This will keep your mind occupied when, left to its own devices, it would gravitate toward thoughts about crystal. Do something interesting with friends rather than stay at home feeling bored, lonely, and sorry for yourself because you otherwise would be out getting high on meth during that time. Other activities may not feel as satisfying at first, and that's alright. However, they will help get you through the rough initial period.

Even after you have made it through the early stages of stopping crystal, sticking to a structured schedule is a basic principle of relapse prevention. Structure prevents boredom, a big trigger for drug use; it keeps your mind occupied when all it wants to think about is crystal; and it helps you feel productive, and positive about yourself. A structured life is the opposite of the addict life, which is organized on whim and the need for immediate gratification. So structure takes you into a healthier lifestyle and gives you a balanced framework that encourages moderation and discipline.

To fill your schedule, think of activities that take you out of the house, such as playing a sport or taking a class in something that has always interested you. Think of people with whom you can spend time in healthy and enjoyable ways. Keep your schedule organized and realistic. Include time for work, exercise, rest, and most important, healthy fun. Balance is the key to making your structure work—it prevents you from burning out. With the correct balance, structure will eventually feels stabilizing and comfortable, not restraining.

REWARD YOURSELF

CALCULATE HOW MUCH money you used to spend on crystal. When totaled up, this can be a shocking amount. Calculate how much money you would have spent on meth in a single month. Make a list of ten different things that you could buy with that amount of money. Pick one of those items on the list as a reward you promise yourself at the end of the month if you stay clean. To make sure this stays an active motivator during the course of the month, set weekly goals for yourself. For example, suppose you used to spend $400 per month on crystal, or approximately $100 per week. At the end of each week that you stick to your sobriety, take $100 and buy a gift card at a store that sells the item that you want to buy. Put the gift cards somewhere visible so you can remind yourself how well you are doing and what kind of reward you are building up to. At the end of one month, you will have $400 in gift cards to purchase the item you want.

The rationale for buying gift cards each week is that you need to have frequent small rewards throughout the month to keep you motivated, and by putting the cash into gift cards, you will not be able to use the money to buy crystal if you are suddenly hit with a strong craving. Many places, such as Starbucks, Sears, Circuit City, major clothing stores, many restaurants, and even nail salons and spas, offer gift cards. Many gift cards can be purchased online, so they are convenient and easy to get.

The concept of a reward incentive may sound childish, like giving a child candy for behaving well. But this is probably why it works—it appeals to the more primitive part of the brain and doesn't require logic or higher brain processing. Research has repeatedly shown that this technique, called contingency management, is one of the most successful interventions to keep addicts clean. A recent study by the National Institute on Drug Abuse found that almost 50 percent of people who were rewarded for drug-free urine fondly called "peeing for prizes," were able to complete a twelve-week treatment program, compared to 35 percent of people who were given only verbal praise. Offering rewards to addicts increased the likelihood that they would be sober at any one time, it quadrupled their chances of remaining completely drug-free for the *entire* twelve weeks of the treatment, and it increased the likelihood that the person would stick with treatment, even if they slipped.

Positron emission tomography (PET) scan shows images of how the brain reacts during different thinking tasks. A study of what parts of the brain are active during states of happiness looked at the brain while subjects focused on different "happy" things. Warm and positive memories about family and childhood activated particular parts of the brain, while money and material goods activated *different* brain centers—the same areas of the brain activated by cocaine and methamphetamine. In addition to the psychological effects of contingency management, there seems to be a biological basis for the efficacy of rewards—they may stimulate brain regions that are impaired and less active after chronic drug use. Gently stimulating these areas with rewards may increase chronically low dopamine activity, satisfying a biological need, and thereby stave off further craving and relapse.

HOW TO TOLERATE CRAVINGS

"CRAVING" REFERS TO both the emotional and physical feelings of wanting to use something. In this book craving refers specifically to crystal, though people can crave other drugs, foods, activities—almost anything. The implication of the word craving is that your desire exists despite the knowledge that you cannot have the thing you want. Cravings vary from mild, passing thoughts about using to intense and overwhelming feelings with bodily reactions, such as tingling skin, rumbling in the stomach, intestinal cramps, and even diarrhea. Cravings can feel irresistible, as if you are compelled to act on them. When craving is intense, you may feel that you have no option, that you *must* use. But no matter how urgent the feeling, if you don't use crystal, you will still be alive the next day. And you'll be much healthier.

This section gives a few suggestions for handling cravings. Thoughts about crystal can cause physiological reactions in your body that occur in conjunction with other types of anxiety. Therefore, some relaxation techniques are often helpful.

Deep Breathing and Muscle Relaxation Exercise

The first time you do this exercise, have a friend read you the instructions as you do the steps. Choose a friend with a calm, relaxing voice who can slowly lead you through each step. After one or two times, you will be able to do this exercise alone from memory. However, if hearing another person giving you soothing instructions feels more effective, have your friend read the instructions on a tape that you can play whenever you do the exercise. Hearing your friend's voice may also be a nice reminder that you are not alone, and that other people care about you and your sobriety.

INSTRUCTIONS:

Find a comfortable and quiet place where you can lie down. Lie on your back, close your eyes, and place your hands at your side. Take a slow, deep breath through your mouth over 5 seconds, then exhale slowly through your nose over 5 seconds. Take 3 deep breaths like this, slowly inhaling and exhaling.

Continue to breathe this way throughout the entire exercise. With time it will feel natural, and you won't even have to think about it.

Tighten your fists, squeezing them as hard as you can. Keep holding them tightly for 5 seconds . . . and relax. When you unclench your fists, focus on the sensation of the blood rushing back into them and feel the tension melt away from your hands.

Next, squeeze your fists in the same way, and press your arms against your sides, pushing them against your body as hard as you can. Hold the position for 5 seconds . . . and relax, again feeling the blood rushing back into your arms and hands as you release the tension. Take a moment for another slow breath in and out.

Now, curl your toes and clench them tightly, together with your fists and your arms. Tighten and hold them all for 5 seconds . . . and relax. Take another slow breath in and out.

Press your knees together, pushing as hard as you can. Now you are squeezing your toes, your knees, your fists, and your arms. Hold the position for 5 seconds . . . and relax. Take another slow breath in and out.

Now, lift your shoulders up toward your head and tense up your neck (skip this step if you have any history of neck injury or pain), tensing up every part of your body and hold the position for 5 seconds—focus your mind on the tension in your fists, your arms, your toes, your knees, and your shoulders. Then relax. Take another slow breath in and out.

Scrunch up your face, tightening your eyes and your mouth as hard as you can. You should be tensing every possible muscle in your body now, squeezing them as hard as you can. Hold for 5 seconds . . . and relax.

Feel the waves of blood flowing back into all your body parts. Focus on the sensations and try to be aware of every part of your body.

Now, imagine that your head, shoulders, arms, and legs are made of lead and are extremely heavy. Feel them sinking into the floor or the cushions under you. Let your shoulders drop as your feel their weight, and relax them as you let them sink into the cushions.

Slowly take 5 more deep breaths. Count backward slowly from 10 to 1. When you reach 1, slowly open your eyes.

The Wave

This exercise deals with urges and cravings by using a relaxation and visualization technique. Sit in a comfortable chair and close your eyes. Take 3 slow, deep breaths, just as you did in the muscle relaxation exercise. Now imagine yourself standing on a beach ankle-deep in the water. Visualize your cravings as a wave that is building up to a crest. The wave may be very high, depending on the intensity of your cravings. Watch the wave come closer, but stay where you are. Do not run away from it. In fact, imagine yourself sitting down in the shallow edge of the water, waiting for the wave to come. When it arrives, it may buffet you with a strong force at first, but sitting in the sand, you are stable and are able to hold your ground. The wave keeps moving and you can feel it wash over your body. Gradually it passes over you and runs past you, disappearing into foam on the beach. Then watch it gradually recede into the ocean, taking your cravings out to sea. Take 3 more deep breaths and slowly open your eyes.

This technique is a relaxation exercise that helps you to conceptualize your physical and psychological cravings in a visual metaphor, the wave. It reminds you that if you stay where you are and just do nothing, the urge will eventually pass. When you have a craving, despite the urgency and desperation you feel, *nothing* will happen if you do not use. You have survived cravings in the past, and you will survive even more in the future. Each time you successfully let a craving pass, the tension will become less intense and the next wave will seem smaller. This is a convenient exercise because it is simple and it can be done whenever you feel a craving, whether you are at home, at work, or sitting on a bus or in the subway.

DEVISING NEW WAYS TO COPE WITH BAD FEELINGS

FOR ADDICTS, DRUGS have become the major way of coping with negative emotions. Even if you do not have immediate access to crystal, just the knowledge that you can get high when you get home may comfort you in a tough situation. Giving up drugs completely takes away your most familiar and comfortable way to ward off bad feelings. Before using drugs, you had other ways of dealing with problems, but after a long time of depending on crystal, you may have forgotten them and will need to relearn them.

If you feel upset, frustrated, sad, or angry, what are some ways that you can deal with your feelings without resorting to crystal or other drugs? Think of answers to this question when your mood is good and you are thinking rationally because when unhappiness suddenly hits you, you will be in no frame of mind to think of good solutions. The more upset you are, the more desperately you will grasp for any way to feel better. Since the most familiar solution to your problems may be crystal, if you have not prepared any alternative plan of action, doing crystal may be the only solution in sight.

Think about what you can do *immediately* when you get upset. What are things that can distract yourself from unpleasant feelings, help you to relax, or help you blow off some steam? One technique is to immediately stop what you are doing and take ten deep breaths while repeating a calming phrase, such as "Everything is all right," or "I am still a good person." Other examples include taking a slow walk around the block to clear your head, doing some exercise like jogging, calling a friend or twelve-step sponsor, taking a long, hot bath, trying one of your relaxation exercises, going to a yoga class, or attending the nearest twelve-step meeting. Make a list with several techniques that you know can soothe you, so that you have a long list of options other than drugs that are possible in any situation.

Also consider *intermediate* interventions that can help you cope. This includes making plans during the week that you can look forward to, so that despite whatever unpleasant event you are going through now, you can expect relief sometime soon. Using intermediate interventions is a way to practice tolerating frustration for short periods of time. You will gradually be able to tolerate longer periods of time without needing immediate gratification and instant relief. Examples include getting regular massages each week, watching a movie or a show, seeing an exhibit at the local museum, or having dinner at your favorite restaurant. Choose realistic activities that you enjoy. Anticipating the enjoyment later in the week can pull you through a difficult situation in the present. When you finally make it to your planned activity, it also feels like a well-deserved reward, which reinforces the success of your new coping skill.

Finally, set up some long-term goals, such as improving your health, furthering your education, moving along in your career, and improving your relationships. Don't pressure yourself too much, but focus your eyes on the horizon. These goals will remind you why it is important not to relapse and will keep your motivation strong. When you are stuck in a bad situation, contemplating your long-term goals will pull you out of your current emotional chaos and give you a broader perspective on your own life. Despite whatever unpleasant thing is happening to you right now, step back and see your life moving in a good direction as you keep working toward your long-term goals. Think of the old sailor's remedy for seasickness—if you keep your sight fixed on the steady horizon in the distance, you will not feel so sick from the rocking of the boat right under your feet.

See exercise 10-3, "Coping Skills," (page 132) to make a list of activities tailored to your personality and needs.

EXERCISE 10-1 IDENTIFYING LIFESTYLE
OR EMOTIONAL ISSUES

WHAT aspects of your life make you automatically think of using crystal?

Think about all areas of your life (general emotional state, job, relationships, sex, family, medical problems, etc.).

_____

_____

_____

_____

_____

_____

_____

_____

_____

_____

_____

EXERCISE 10-2 IDENTIFYING HIGH-RISK SITUATIONS

MAKE a list of people, places, and things that remind you of using crystal:

People:

_____

_____

_____

_____

_____

Places:

_____

_____

_____

_____

_____

Things:

_____

_____

_____

_____

_____

EXERCISE 10-3 COPING SKILLS

Use to:

- Develop more adaptive immediate self-soothing techniques
- Develop & strengthen your ability to tolerate frustration over time (intermediate and long-term strategies)
- Remind yourself of long-term goals to put immediate problems into perspective and to build your self-esteem

List five things you can do immediately (today) to make yourself feel better (e.g., hot shower, take a walk in the park):

1.

2.

3.

4.

5.

List five things you can do this week to make yourself feel better (e.g., go to a museum, get a massage):

1.

2.

3.

4.

5.

List five things you can do in the future that will make your life more satisfying (e.g., improve your relationships, go back to school, advance in your career, cut down the stressful things in your life):

1.

2.

3.

4.

5.

11

THINGS YOU CAN DO TO BEAT CRYSTAL ADDICTION:
Some Specific Strategies

CHAPTER **10** DISCUSSED the general principles of relapse prevention. This chapter will look at specific activities that can help you move forward along the road to a drug-free life. All the activities discussed follow the guiding principles of relapse prevention: understanding and avoiding risky situations and learning to cope with the unavoidable.

TALK ABOUT IT

TALK WITH PEOPLE about your experiences with crystal. Find a person that you trust, someone with whom you feel safe sharing this information. Talking about drugs with sober friends and family may not be comfortable— if it were easy, you would have done it already. Possible people include your partner or spouse; a family member; a friend who knows you well, even if you have not spoken with that friend for a long while. Whoever you chose, be sure the person *does not use drugs*. Former drug users who are in successful recovery can be extremely helpful because they have been in your shoes—they can understand the highs and the lows you've felt on meth, as well as the difficulty of your current struggle. People who have never tried crystal are also helpful, but they must be open-minded, without automatically condemning you for your past drug use. They can listen to your story with a thoughtful ear, offer you compassion and support, and remind you what your own life was like before crystal, which may seem like a completely different person's life. The process of explaining your drug history and your feelings to someone drug-naïve, trying to get them to understand what it was like, may actually help you clarify your own thoughts. Whoever you choose—a former meth user, someone in recovery from other drugs, or someone who's never tried drugs—will have something to offer if you open up to them. The more people you can talk with, the better. When temptations are strong, they can support you through difficult times, when you might otherwise be led to relapse.

Open yourself up and be honest. Whoever you speak with needs to hear *everything*, both the good and the bad experiences: your feelings, desires, and fears of *using* crystal, as well as your feelings, desires, and fears of *stopping*. To benefit from talking with others, you should end the conversation feeling understood. While it is rare to find someone who can understand you completely, if you feel the other person can't see the picture at all, find someone else. Do not let the frustration of feeling misunderstood grow into a rationalization to use again. On the other hand, if people respond with words that don't sit quite right with you, before disagreeing or trying to correct them, try to keep your ears open and examine what they are saying. This follows the AA adage "Take the cotton out of your ears and put it in your mouth." Before you say anything, take a minute to ponder their words, consider if this completely different point of view may have anything that might be relevant to you, and then give your response. You may be so used to your old view of your drug use and sobriety that new ideas that initially sound completely off the mark may actually be right on target.

Sharing the fact that you are addicted can lift a tremendous burden off your shoulders. Holding such a big secret creates tremendous pressure, and the tension creates a wall that separates you from your family and friends. Opening up to people about your addiction allows you to connect with them in an honest way. Lying and hiding are survival skills in the drug-using world. In time, they weave their way into an addict's life so completely that, after a while, they become a part of every interaction, even when there is no reason to hide the truth. At that point, the addict may be unable to connect with anyone in an honest and sincere way.

An interesting note to add here is that while crystal makes your brain think you are happy, psychologists have found that one of the strongest determinants of "happiness" is meaningful interpersonal connections, which are usually lost when people become severely addicted to crystal. So reestablish those connections, and don't listen to the addicted brain telling you that you'll never feel happy without crystal. Staying clean and improving interpersonal connections may be the best way to recover *true* happiness.

By talking about your addiction to others, you are constantly reminding yourself. The addicted part of you wants to deny any problem with crystal, even if it has completely destroyed your life, and that desire to deny will always be lurking, waiting for you to believe it. The moment you let your guard down, the lurking addict takes the opportunity to trick you, concocting an innocent excuse to try crystal again: "It's been four years without crystal, and I can't remember the last time I even thought about it. Everyone is going to be partying tonight, so what's the harm in doing just one bump? After four years, I should be fine."

Sharing the story of your addiction with others makes it real. It is like the old question, "If a tree falls in the forest and no one is there to hear it, does it make a sound?" Make sure someone else hears your admission. The tree fell, and you both heard it, so you know it made a sound—you both know that you have an addiction, and it is real. Down the road, when you may feel weak, it will be harder to deny the past so that you can rationalize using again. This is another step toward successful recovery.

If you still can't talk about your addiction with anybody, ask yourself why not. The addict side of you may be rationalizing and making any possible excuse to avoid things that would help you quit. This is a cardinal sign of addiction: despite knowing you need to stop using, you can't control the part of your brain that still wants to use—rather, that part controls you. Fighting that part of your brain is difficult, so enlist the help of others. This is another important reason that talking with others will help you overcome the addictive forces in your mind.

Research shows that the more social support one has—the more friends and family who are aware and supportive of the recovery—the better the chances of becoming controlling the addiction. There are many possible reasons for this, though nobody knows the definitively. Whatever the reason, the numbers speak for themselves. Involving friends and family in your recovery helps—a lot.

INDIVIDUAL COUNSELING

IN ADDITION TO talking with friends and family, working with a professional who specializes in addiction is a crux of early treatment. In the past, "drug treatment" consisted of an addict simply listening to admonitions or instructions from a health care provider. This was a passive process. The addict was a "patient" who expected to be cured on hearing the magical words from an insightful healer. However, nothing magical about the doctor elicits a cure, and a passive attitude will doom an addict to relapse. This antiquated method of addiction treatment needed a complete overhaul.

Recovery is an active process that requires hard work. You and your counselor should work together as a team toward a goal that you set out for yourself: it is *your* addiction, it is *your* recovery, and it is *your* responsibility, hard work, and sweat that will keep you sober. Ultimately, you are the driver of this car. Drug counselors sit in the passenger seat next to you. They point out helpful landmarks along the road, and they suggest driving techniques that will keep you safely on the right course. In real terms, counselors use their experience with addicts to help you understand your addiction more fully, alert you when your addictive side starts to act up, and lend you their experience in coping with the difficulties of recovery.

An effective counselor must have experience working with addicts, recognizing addictive behaviors, and being familiar with skills to cope with cravings. A counselor needs to be supportive and empathic but also needs to confront you when you veer toward drug thinking. Confrontation is usually uncomfortable, and if you become defensive, it can seem downright offensive. A defensive reaction tells you, "This person doesn't know what I'm going through and has no respect for me!" But counselors are actually being empathic with the part of you that wants to stop crystal, the part of you that is asking for help. They are showing you tremendous respect by believing that the sober part of you is strong enough to succeed. The counselor's job is to point to subtle signs that addictive behavior may be sneaking back into control.

If your counselor says something that makes you angry, think again of that AA expression "Take the cotton out of your ears and stick it in your mouth." Stop the automatic impulse to argue back, try to open your mind, and ask yourself what is making you so upset. If you search really hard, you may see that your addict side is yelling back because it feels threatened. If this is so, your counselor may be doing excellent work—making your addict side feel so threatened means that your hard work is paying off and the addict side is losing control.

While having a drug counselor experienced with crystal is ideal, many areas still lack health care professionals who are very knowledgeable about meth. Nonetheless, a general drug counselor can still be helpful. The principles of recovery apply to all addictions, regardless of the specific drug. Crystal-specific knowledge can provide additional benefit, but if it's not available, don't turn away from the valuable resource that you do have. Take the opportunity to learn the basics of addiction recovery.

Some of you may find that you know more about meth than your drug counselor, and you may have to teach him or her a few things about the drug. Avoid the assumption that this person is therefore unable to help you. The fundamental problems of all addictions are the same, and you need someone who understands addictive behaviors and has experience in helping people overcome them.

If you are already seeing a psychotherapist who was not aware of your crystal addiction, and now you need to work on sobriety, you should keep the focus of your sessions on achieving sobriety and learning relapse prevention skills before moving back to the other life issues you usually discuss in your therapy. While it may be tempting to talk about your troubled childhood that led to your difficulty with relationships today, you need to shelve that important topic for later. There are three reasons for this:

Most important, you need to devote all your mental energy to getting off crystal and learning specific skills, which you need now to cope without crystal. It takes tremendous work, so take it seriously, and devote the time to it that it deserves. Your brain is in the physiological grip of a strong chemical addiction that supersedes logical thinking. While understanding the childhood experiences that may have led you to addiction are important, that understanding is not helpful now. Stopping crystal and learning how to keep off the drug are more pressing at this time.

In addition, exploring life issues in therapy can increase distress. Exploratory therapy, as opposed to relapse-prevention therapy" usually causes emotional discomfort as you uncover buried issues—your mind originally buried them because it was too uncomfortable for you to keep them at a conscious level. In long-term therapy, uncovering issues is necessary in order to examine and address them. However, this is a long-term process. When you are first trying to achieve sobriety, adding additional stress just when you are trying to stay away from drugs can make you fall right back into them. At this time, you should focus on developing skills to protect yourself from uncomfortable feelings and avoid exploring things that will make you more upset and fall back on your most familiar coping mechanism, crystal. Once your skills at handling difficult feelings without drugs are stronger, then it will be time to go back to exploratory therapy. In the long run, understanding these roots of your character my help your addiction, in addition to the rest of you life.

Finally, issues other than sobriety may *seem* important in therapy, but they may just be distractions created by the sneaky addicted part of your brain, trying to divert your attention away from sobriety. The insidious addict in you may try to convince you, "If only I could resolve my troubles in this one particular relationship, then I wouldn't need crystal anymore." Meanwhile, focusing all of your sessions on the ups and downs of your relationship rather than developing skills to stop meth leaves you vulnerable to keep using. The addict in you quietly hopes that this tactic can buy you months to years more of crystal use before you and your therapist realize that therapy has just been going in circles, while your addiction to meth has gotten worse. Wait until you have acquired the skills to face stress without relapsing. Then you are ready to work on other life issues safely.

TWELVE-STEP PROGRAMS

Twelve-step programs are probably best known by their earliest incarnation, **Alcoholics Anonymous** (AA). This group was designed as a "spiritual" way of dealing with addiction by Bill Wilson (known in AA as Bill W.), a Wall Street market analyst, and Dr. Robert Smith (known in AA as Dr. Bob). Both Bill W. and Dr. Bob had been active alcoholics. Bill W. had been through multiple treatments and attempts to stay sober, at times being told that he was a hopeless case because of his repeated relapses. In 1935, Bill W. and Dr. Bob met each other, and during their long discussions about their mutual addictions, they experienced something new. Telling one's experience and sharing it openly with someone who validated it from his own personal experience was something that neither of them had ever encountered in the past, either in the medical system or religious communities. That moment is considered the birth of the original AA. Since its meager beginnings with a small group of alcoholics gathering in Akron, Ohio, AA has now grown to more than 2 million members, with more than 100,000 groups in over 150 countries.

Originally AA was heavily influenced by religion and incorporated a Christian-centered devotion to God; however, the fundamental ideas have been useful to people of all religious or nonreligious backgrounds, and AA groups are successful in non-Christian countries, such as Cambodia, Israel, and Dubai.*

The following are important concepts that address the core issues of addiction:

1. Admission that one has an addiction.
2. Admission that one is powerless against the addiction.
3. Submission to the powerlessness.
4. Reaching out for help from others.

Addicts usually do not recognize, or will not admit, that they have a problem, often until it is too late. Even when meth addicts suspect that their use is growing beyond their control, they keep themselves in denial, and so are reluctant to talk about crystal as if it were a problem. As they try to hold on to the fantasy that they still have control, their addiction grows stronger. A key concept of twelve-step programs, which is echoed several times in this book, is the ability to "let go." Addicts teach themselves through repeated drug use that they can "control" their world. When something does not feel right, there is always a pill, a drink, or another drug that can make them feel better. The fact that crystal users often know more about the drug than many physicians reinforces their conviction that they know better than anyone else what they need, and that they can control everything in their lives. This is one of the biggest obstacles that addicts face, and it is the *first* of the twelve steps: admitting one is powerless and letting go of the control.

*In the United States, depending on which meeting you attend, the language of the group may still have a heavily Christian feel, but belief in a Christian God is *not* an essential part of the current AA philosophy. If one group seems too extreme in its religious orientation for your comfort, try another, and hopefully you will find one that is a better fit.

Another powerful aspect of twelve-step programs is the fellowship with other people who have the same addiction, i.e., finding a group of people who really *understand* you. Speaking with other crystal users in recovery is powerful. You hear the words of other people who have experienced the strong grip of this addiction—the amazing highs, the nightmare crashes, the irresistible lure of the drug, and the gradual destruction it can cause in your life as you watch things fall apart, unable to resist the draw to use it again. People who've never tried meth can only try to imagine what you've experienced, whereas these people *know* because they have been there. At twelve-step meetings you hear other people tell stories similar to yours, and you have the opportunity to share your experiences and receive support from understanding peers. Telling your stories, good or bad, can inspire others to stay clean, and hearing the tragic stories of others may give you more motivation to stay clean.

The benefit of peer-led groups goes beyond empathy and support. Because people in the groups have been in your position, not only do they share the addiction and the desire for sobriety, they also share the experience of relapsing. They can see if your life is veering in a dangerous direction—overloading yourself with stress or unrealistic expectations, repeating behaviors that have gotten you into trouble with crystal before, or rationalizing and allowing dangerous triggers of meth back into your life. Peers can confront you and "call you on your B.S." with a convincing authority that non–crystal users can never have. It is much easier to ignore the advice of someone who does not know what it is like to be hooked on crystal. However, when the same words come from another addict in recovery, they may shake you up enough to actually stop and listen.

Every new member of a twelve-step program finds a "sponsor," a senior member with a substantial length of sobriety to whom the new member can look for support and mentorship. The sponsor is supposed to be available whenever the new member is feeling weak, trying to fight off cravings. Rather than reach for a drug, the member can reach for the phone, and often, speaking with the sponsor helps to abort a potential relapse.

Twelve-step groups now exist for all types of addiction, even non-drug addictions, such as addictions to food and sex. When **Crystal Meth Anonymous** (CMA) was first formed, there were few meetings, and those were poorly attended. Now in most major cities, CMA meetings are plentiful and often packed to standing-room capacity. Clearly there is a need for even more CMA meetings, as existing meetings are over capacity; in many towns, CMA meetings don't yet exist. For specific information about the closest CMA meetings to you, visit the Web site www.crystalmeth.org, which frequently updates lists of meeting locations and times throughout the country. Fortunately, the list of CMA meetings continues to grow to try to meet the expanding need.

Many people underestimate the power of peer-led support groups such as CMA and AA. Initially the medical community was extremely skeptical about twelve-step groups, with many physicians feeling that addicts getting advice from other addicts was like the blind leading the blind. However, studies have shown the tremendous impact of twelve-step meetings. A study by McKellar and colleagues in 2003, and another by Moos and Moos in 2004, demonstrated that people who were more involved in AA were more likely to be sober than those less involved, and this effect persisted up to eight years from the time of joining AA. Another study by McKellar, Stewart, and Humphries in 2003 looked at the effect of attending AA in a group of 2,319 men in the Veterans Affairs hospital system. Interestingly, motivation to be sober and belief in the AA program itself had no correlation with success. Even those reporting low motivation stayed in recovery longer if they continued to attend AA meetings.

Even if you are doing other things to try to address your crystal addiction, attending a twelve-step program can still be extremely helpful. A study by Timko and colleagues in 2000 showed that people who added twelve-step groups to "traditional" addiction treatment more than doubled their rate of staying clean, and they had maintained this benefit when they were followed up three years later.

The message is that peer-led twelve-step meetings are helpful, and statistically speaking, even if you don't like them, they significantly increase your chances of staying clean. Without an answer to *how* or *why* they work, for whatever reason, they are associated with a better outcome, which is what matters most.

CRYSTAL METH ANONYMOUS (CMA)—THE GOOD AND THE BAD

PEER-LED SUPPORT groups should be part of any recovery program, in addition to your own personal efforts, individual counseling, medications, or whatever else you find helpful. In addition to the concepts discussed above, the anonymity of these organizations is crucial. Some meetings are "open" to anyone who would like to come. Others are "closed" meetings, only for people who are established CMA members. There is an implicit understanding that CMA, and all other twelve-step groups, are completely confidential. What happens in "the walls," referring to the meetings, stays within the walls, and identities are never revealed outside. The safety of the anonymity is crucial to allow you to feel as free as possible to open up and be as honest as you can to yourself, as well as to others.

Because CMA meetings are relatively new and pockets of the crystal-using community in major cities are relatively concentrated, CMA meetings do not always feel anonymous. Even in large cities, such as New York and Los Angeles, you may recognize many faces—people in your social circle or people you may have even hooked up with on the Internet or at sex parties. On the one hand, this can be a good thing. Seeing familiar faces strongly reinforces the message that you are not alone. You can already see this by the crowd of people at many of the meetings. However, seeing people that you already know in your life drives the point home. Maybe you thought that among your group of crystal buddies, you were the only one with a problem. However, by seeing them at CMA, you know that you are not the only one struggling with meth addiction.

On the other hand, when people are still too afraid to let their friends or family know about their crystal use, seeing familiar faces can create more fear than reassurance. In that case, the chance of seeing people you know may deter you from ever visiting a CMA meeting. In that case, try an AA group or a **Narcotics Anonymous** (NA) group first. All twelve-step groups use the same principles, though the flavor and the stories may vary a little. At the beginning, the most important task is to join a group of peers with whom you feel comfortable who share the determination to be sober. Even with AA and NA meetings, it usually requires attending several different groups to find one that feels comfortable for you. After developing more strength in your conviction to stay clean and less shame about your addiction, it may matter less that you recognize people at CMA, and if it is helpful, you can try to attend a CMA meeting again. Because it is specific to your drug of choice, you will hear stories and can share experiences that you may relate to more strongly. For example, crystal can give people uncontrollable, intense sexual experiences that are difficult for nonusers to understand. Sharing one's difficulties and getting advice about dealing with sex may be easier at CMA meetings. But decide whatever feels best for you.

Even if you decide you are comfortable with CMA, recognize that not every CMA meeting is appropriate for every individual. Again, find the meeting that feels like the best fit for you. For example, if you are newly sober and you are looking for role models and success stories to inspire you, then groups with only new members may overload you with too many stories of vicious struggles with sobriety and frequent relapses. Also, seeing recent crystal-sex partners in meetings may be a strong a trigger rather than a source of support. Some meetings may feel like people are coming just to pick up someone for crystal sex. The unfortunate reality is that it happens. If you find this, go to another meeting. If the members of one meeting are so different from you that you find it difficult to relate, try another group. Now there are enough meetings that groups have taken on different flavors, and you have more of a choice. If that's not yet the case where you live, try AA meetings, which, because of their long history, have a much wider variety from which to choose.

One of my patients working on alcohol addiction was an upper-middle-class former beauty pageant winner in her midforties. Initially she insisted on attending meetings with people whom she described as "totally down-and-out." Many of the members were homeless, and some were schizophrenic. She rationalized that seeing how badly addiction could affect people would motivate her to stay sober. However, in reality she used the dramatic difference between her and the group members to convince herself that she was not nearly as addicted as the others in the group, so was not open to their support, and she convinced herself that she did not really have any problem with addiction. She relapsed very quickly. After detoxing, she found it was much more difficult for her to attend groups with people who were similar to her because she had to confront her own addiction more directly—at those meetings, she could see different aspects of herself in the other people in the room. This was frightening at the beginning, but eventually she was better able to admit her own addiction, and eventually she was able to accept both her own illness and the support and advice of people in the group because they were more similar to her.

Unfortunately, some places have very few CMA, AA, NA, or other twelve-step meetings. In this case, you may not have the luxury of choosing from a long list of meetings to attend. Finding the best fit is optimal, just like choosing the right-size coat. However, even the wrong-size coat may give you some protection from the cold. In the same way, you may still benefit from a twelve-step program with people who are not exactly like you. At least give the twelve-step meetings a try, and attend at least five different meetings before you give up and say there's no possibility of getting any help from these groups. The other pieces in your recovery program, such as a drug counselor, can help you look for useful elements in the groups. However, do not let yourself fall into the trap of rationalizing, like the patient I described. Describe the group and discuss your reactions with an addiction professional to discern whether the group has any beneficial or potentially harmful effects on you. If you are clear on its limitations, you may still be able to benefit from a group that isn't exactly a perfect fit.

INTENSIVE OUTPATIENT PROGRAMS

IF YOU ARE having trouble staying clean despite working regularly with an individual counselor and going to twelve-step meetings, you may need a higher level of treatment. Intensive outpatient programs (IOPs) that address addictions are the next step up. Usually IOPs consist of a more intensive and structured schedule of individual counseling, support groups, education about drugs and addiction, and twelve-step meetings. The frequency and intensity of the activities vary, and programs are usually tailored to each person's needs. Some people require daily treatment to keep themselves away from crystal and some just go a few days a week. Some people's daily treatment eventually trim down their participation to only two or three evenings each week, which keeps them in a structured program while they integrate back into their day jobs.

CRYSTAL-SPECIFIC TREATMENT PROGRAMS

WHILE THE MAJORITY of IOPs are general and include people with addictions to all kinds of drugs, a program designed specifically for the needs of crystal users would be even more helpful to you. This makes intuitive sense, because crystal-specific programs focus more attention on the problems that are most common for meth users.

Let's take gay male crystal users as an example. Some closeted gay men were first introduced to the gay community in the setting of nightclubs and circuit parties, where many of these men were first able to feel comfortable and excited about their sexuality, rather than ashamed. In these settings, club drugs such as Ecstasy, ketamine, GHB, cocaine, and crystal were commonly used, and drug use in these places was the norm. For these men, crystal, as well as the use of other club drugs, was attached to the joyously liberating experience of coming out and finally feeling free about their sexuality. For these men, the emotional meaning of crystal is much more complicated than just feeling high or enjoying sex. Rather, crystal is also associated with life-changing memories of finally accepting oneself and one's own sexuality, and by using drugs, these men were able to bond with a like-minded community. Mourning the loss of the intense high that crystal gives is difficult by itself. But these men are also being forced to reject a social scene with strong emotional meaning. And for those whose social network is still primarily drug-using club-goers, the very people who made them feel accepted—how will they turn their backs on them? And without them, will they be as isolated and alone as they had been before coming out? Again, Nancy Reagan's Just Say No campaign oversimplifies the complexity of addiction. The act of quitting a drug needs to be fully explored to help people quit. In this case, these gay men needed to find healthier ways to accept their sexuality, find healthier peers, and improve their self-esteem.

The example of gay male crystal users is only one of many. Every type of crystal user—from teenage girls with eating disorders to young men in the rural South, struggling with boredom and low self-worth—has a story that needs to be explored, and their underlying vulnerabilities need to be addressed specifically, as well, to reduce the chances of their turning back to crystal.

Finding Mutual Support BRIAN'S STORY

When Brian, a lawyer, was discharged from the hospital, he went directly to a residential drug-addiction treatment facility that specializes in crystal addiction. He explored his gay identity and the significance of his connection to the gay community through clubs and drugs. He wrestled with a tremendous fear of giving up this part of his life and feelings of guilt for turning his back on the social group that finally allowed him to accept himself as a gay man. His fellow circuit partyers were his family. The entire social scene surrounding his use of crystal was extremely important to him. Trying to convince him to "avoid people, places, and things" to completely kick the drug and everything that came with it was much harder than he had imagined.

Sex was another intensive focus in Brian's groups. In other programs, he felt that non–meth users had no idea what crystal-sex was like, and they didn't comprehend the intensity of the compulsive need to feed his turbocharged libido, or the disappointing emptiness of sex without crystal. In this group, the members started from a point of common understanding. There was mutual support, but in addition, the group worked on specific strategies for dealing with sex: understanding the different components of sex, realistic expectations about sex in the future, mourning the loss of crystal-sex, and exercises to relearn aspects of sex that were lost when he was using crystal. Mourning crystal sex continues to be a struggle, but Brian felt more hopeful, glad that he was actively working on something important to him rather than simply being told, "That's terrible, but everything will get better with time."

After Brian finished his inpatient rehabilitation, he continued to go to CMA meetings, where he was surprised to find other people he had seen at circuit parties and sex clubs. Some had been sober for over a year, and some who recently joined were going through a lot of the same early struggles that Brian had experienced. In groups with gay men who were just recently clean, he was able to give and receive mutual support. However, at times Brian found those groups difficult because they stirred up old memories and triggers. Many of the newly sober men kept relapsing, and some openly invited Brian to have sex with crystal. Fortunately he was smart enough to change to an early-morning group, with other professional men who were more like Brian. They were motivated to stop because they had long, successful careers that were in jeopardy. Brian's law firm was still unaware of his drug-use problem—he was extremely discreet and paid for all his treatment with his own savings. He never filed health insurance claims, and he used vacation and sick leave to take time off from work for his rehab. Brian watched some of his crystal buddies who had also been successful professionals in their late thirties lose their jobs, lose their professional licenses, and move back in with their parents as if they were teenagers. He knew his job was on the line, and after working so long to be an attorney, he was determined not to let crystal take away everything he had worked for.

Men and women who used crystal primarily during sex often fear that sex will never be enjoyable without crystal. Sex itself becomes a tremendous trigger to use again. For human beings, sex is a natural desire that will always be there. How do these people cope? Do they ever have that level of pleasurable sex again? These questions need to be discussed because the issue of sex will never go away and cannot be ignored—it is one of the toughest aspects of crystal addiction. What are some coping skills to handle sex during the early stages of recovery? How can one relearn how to have sober sex and enjoy it? A comprehensive treatment program identifies these areas and teaches skills to cope with problems as well as exercises that may improve these areas. In this example, sex is the issue, but for others, the issue may be body image, self-esteem, stress management, and self-expectations. Specific topics, when effectively addressed in a supportive environment, have been shown to improve abstinence rates for crystal addicts.

THE MATRIX MODEL

A CRYSTAL-SPECIFIC program addresses the examples above as well as others in focused support and educational groups. One of the earliest models of crystal-focused treatment is the **Matrix Model**, developed by a group of addiction specialists at UCLA. The Matrix Model is an intensive treatment program based on traditional relapse-prevention concepts, with a specific focus on methamphetamine.

Large-scale studies comparing crystal addicts in Matrix Model programs with crystal addicts in treatment-as-usual (TAU) programs found that crystal-specific treatment kept people engaged in treatment longer, reduced the number of relapses (verified by regular urine drug tests), and helped addicts to sustain longer periods of complete sobriety. Although *both* types of programs showed improvement, those in the crystal-focused program improved significantly more.

A follow-up study of subjects one year after completing intensive treatment found that the advantages of the crystal-focused programs gradually disappeared, and all the patients, regardless of the type of IOP treatment they received, looked identical as far as relapsing. Any advantage that the Matrix Model had initially provided was lost. While crystal-specific IOPs have a clear advantage over TAU, more crystal-specific services at all levels of care are necessary to provide lasting benefits following IOP programs.

INPATIENT OR RESIDENTIAL REHABILITATION

MANY PEOPLE ARE familiar with the concept of twenty-eight-day treatment programs, made well known to the general public by the movie *28 Days,* starring Sandra Bullock. This inpatient form of addiction treatment is used when people have already tried to stop using crystal several times but, no matter how hard they try, they continue to relapse, and they begin to face increasingly dangerous consequences—problems with their health, their job, their relationships, or other important aspects of their lives. Depending on where the program is located, it can be an **inpatient program,** meaning that it is physically located within a hospital, or it can be a **residential program,** which is a freestanding facility without other hospital services. Residential programs are often located in secluded environments, where addicts can peacefully focus on recovery..

Inpatient and residential treatments, as with all other addiction treatments, work best when addicts can admit to their illness and are motivated to stop using crystal. However, even when people lack *complete* insight into their illness, these treatments can still be helpful. This situation of ambivalence and limited insight most often occurs when a person is pressured into treatment by family and friends during an intervention, or if a criminal court mandates that someone receive intensive inpatient or residential drug treatment.

Inpatient treatments remove addicts from their usual environments. Removing as many triggers as possible—the people, places or things that they associate with crystal use—reduces the intensity of their cravings, and they are better able to focus on treatment.

In a controlled setting, access to meth is extremely difficult, so despite any urges to use, addicts are physically unable to relapse as long as they remain in the program. Sometimes breaking the cycle of use, getting completely through the crash, and simply reexperiencing sober thinking again helps tremendously to clear their perspective about the effects of addiction on their lives. During both the high and the crash, addicts' thinking is impaired, and their judgment is affected by extremely strong cravings. Forcing themselves to clean up in a protected, drug-free environment gives addicts a much better start on recovery.

The intensity of inpatient treatment gently but firmly confronts meth addicts and forces them to look at how the drug controls them and how it has affected their lives. Optimally, this is done in a supportive way, because harsh confrontation is usually met with strong resistance and denial—the addict just becomes more adamant that he or she has no problem with drugs. However, through a more gradual process of working through education, self-examination, and learning from other addicts, many skeptical people leave inpatient rehabilitation with improved insight into their addiction, and, it is hoped they have internalized some of the skills to help them stay in recovery.

The actual length of stay at these programs is not necessarily twenty-eight days. Each program sets its own standard, and within each program, the length of stay usually is determined by the severity of each person's addiction. Often, insurance plans will partially cover the expense of a rehabilitation stay. Rehab facilities can vary from low-cost city hospitals to expensive spa-like retreats in secluded or exotic locations. Cosmetics aside, all good programs should have the same basic treatment strategies:

- Individual counseling to closely address personal needs
- Support groups
- Educational groups that teach about crystal and addiction
- Twelve-step meetings

- Teaching skills to manage stress without drugs
- Teaching skills to cope with cravings
- Teaching drug-refusal skills
- Exploration of the family of origin, examination of family dynamics, and active participation of the family and other close supporters in the treatment
- Establishing a plan for how to manage life after leaving program, including connecting you with a drug counselor or therapist, psychiatrist, outpatient program, or whatever is determined to be necessary to maintain the benefit from residential treatment

If you look for inpatient or residential care, make sure that all of these treatments issues are addressed. In addition, make sure that any program you are considering is certified by the **Substance Abuse and Mental Health Services Administration** (SAMHSA), a U.S. government agency that ensures that programs meet or exceed the standards of care set by its state government. This means that the program has been approved by the local state alcohol and drug abuse authority as a substance abuse treatment facility and has responded to the most recent annual National Survey of Substance Abuse Treatment Services. *Be wary of programs that are not accredited.* While they are usually cheaper, this is because they cut corners in necessary treatment modalities and medical supervision. Spending money on a program that does not offer effective clinical treatment is a tremendous waste and risks turning you off to trying other treatment programs that may benefit you greatly. Visit the SAMHSA Web site at http://dasis3.samhsa.gov. You can also contact SAMHSA's Office of Communications by telephone at 240-276-2130, or e-mail info@samhsa.gov.

Another important accrediting organization is the Joint Commission on Accreditation of Healthcare Organizations (JCAHO), a private, not-for-profit organization that assesses thousands of healthcare facilities. If you are considering a program that administers medical treatment, then make sure that it has been certified by JCAHO, which requires strict standards that every medical facility should meet. The emphasis of JCAHO has been on ensuring patients' rights and safety, though to some extent, it also evaluates how well a program meets its clinical goals. Because JCAHO does not specialize in addiction, accreditation from SAMHSA will ensure your medical safety and the quality of your addiction treatment. You can contact

JCAHO by mailing their headquarters at One Renaissance Boulevard, Oakbrook Terrace, IL 60181, or by calling their main telephone number, (630) 792-5000. Visit their Web site at www.jointcommission.org for further information and to check if a program you are considering has been accredited by JCAHO.

Over the past few years, several addiction programs have sprouted up, specifically addressing the treatment of addiction to crystal meth. This is fortunate, because, as research shows, crystal-specific treatment has been shown to have better results. However, some of these new programs and facilities are simply opportunistic, exploiting the devastating health problem of meth addiction. They may offer treatment that is not based on any proven methods or have counselors and clinician's who are not qualified to help you. Therefore, be wary of large for-profit organizations reaching out to you with magazine ads and billboards—they may be more interested in your dollars than in providing you the best help possible. If such a program looks appealing, check with SAMHSA and JCAHO or your state's drug and alcohol treatment services administration to make sure that an advertised program is legitimate.

How do you know if an inpatient rehabilitation program is right for you? Here are some practical guidelines:

1. Have you been completely unable to stop using crystal, despite several attempts at throwing it all away and trying to stay away from triggers?
2. Have you already tried going to CMA meetings and seeing a drug counselor or a therapist experienced with addiction, but you still keep relapsing?
3. Are you having significant medical or psychiatric problems because of crystal use, e.g., possible heart or lung problems, dental problems ("meth-mouth"), episodes of paranoia or hallucinations, severe depression, or suicidal thoughts, but you continue to use?
4. Have you tried intensive outpatient drug programs but they have not been enough to get you to stop using?

If you answered yes to one or more of these questions, then you should consider inpatient treatment. If you answered yes to question 4, then you definitely need more intensive treatment in an inpatient or residential setting.

Many private and group health insurance programs cover some addiction treatment, Usually the most important requirement for insurance coverage is documented failure in outpatient treatment. Ask your insurance company whether it covers inpatient treatment and what the criteria are, because the definition of failing outpatient treatment is arbitrary—it could mean relapsing after seeing a therapist weekly and going to CMA, or it may require a trial of an IOP before inpatient care is even considered. Significant medical or psychiatric illness resulting from drug use will also strongly support your case for coverage.

Unfortunately, most insurance companies are difficult to navigate, and when you are struggling with an illness, it is even harder to negotiate the system. If you are working with a therapist or counselor, ask for help getting through the insurance maze. You can also ask for assistance from your doctor's office manager, a family member, a friend, or a coworker.

Self-Esteem Takes Many Years to Build ANA'S STORY

At first, Ana had a very difficult time with treatment. She was sent to a drug-treatment facility for teens, where she met other teenagers who didn't want treatment but who were also forced by the court or by their parents to be there. She had little insight into her own addiction, and she saw no problem with meth, viewing it as a successful way to be thinner and prettier. Even worse, she blamed her withdrawal symptoms of depression, irritability, and hunger on the program staff, using this as evidence that she was correct in her use of the meds. The doctors' advice to stop meth had only made her feel worse. Ana began hanging out with the teens who were the rebels of the program. Some of them were disruptive in group, speaking up only to ridicule the group or challenge the group leader. Ana was one of a handful of girls who just sat silently, staring angrily at the floor and refusing to contribute to the discussion. After a week, when the irritable depression of her crash began to wane, Ana began to listen to some of the teens who spoke constructively in the group. Although she had originally been angry and had resented the teens who "shared," she started to hear some of what they were saying. Once in a while she heard things she strongly identified with, things she had thought nobody else understood.

Ana made friends with Karen, a sixteen-year-old middle-class Caucasian from San Diego, who had also been trying to lose weight and never felt that she was pretty enough. She understood exactly what Karen meant when she shared in group her frustration with her parents and other adults who she felt had never taken her seriously when she'd complained about how competitive and vicious her high-school classmates could be. Crystal not only made her thinner than her classmates (and prettier, she believed), it also made her feel more confident, immune to the catty stares from the "princesses" in her class. She loved the way the drug made her feel so much better about herself, but she dreaded when its effects would wear off. At times, she saw how trapped she was in using crystal to survive high school, but it was a jungle, and she needed a way to survive. Karen spent most of her time focused on getting more meth. Even when she was feeling anxious and irritable from getting high, she still wanted to keep doing it.

Karen told the group that on meth, she had been gradually deteriorating: one day she passed out in a shopping mall from dehydration and malnutrition. An ambulance brought her to the hospital, and a social worker transferred her directly to this addiction treatment unit. She would never have come on her own. But now that she had been in the program for three weeks, she was beginning to look back on her life with crystal through clearer eyes. Although she had put on weight, her face was still gaunt, and without the rosy glasses of meth she saw in the mirror how sickly she had become. Finally she saw in her own reflection the ugly side of what crystal had done to her.

Karen's story was so familiar to Ana, even though she was one of this girls whom Ana would have resented at her own school in L.A. She was surprised how similar she felt. Here, someone that she would have envied for seeming "perfect" was talking about her own weaknesses and fears, which were identical to Ana's. The sense of connection seemed to give Ana permission and courage to open up about her own feelings, and she began to share her own experiences in groups. She distanced herself from the rebellious teens and began to focus more on trying to feel bet-ter about herself. Without crystal to magically transform her, she had to work hard at changing her feelings, Even though this was a slower, harder process, Ana realized that crystal was only a mask she hid behind to look pretty, but she was the only one fooled by the mask.

Ana worked hard in her rehab program, making gradual progress. Self-esteem, people told her, was something that would take years for her to build, and for many it would be a lifelong process. There were plenty of times when Ana longed for crystal because she remembered the quick relief it gave her. She craved meth the most when she was feeling tired, frustrated, or unattractive. Luckily she was in a protected environment, and she learned to talk to Karen when she really wanted to use. That helped some.

After six weeks, Ana finished the program and returned to her family in L.A. in the middle of that summer. She went to teen AA meetings and stayed sober, keeping in contact with Karen as her "sober sister." However, in the fall, when she returned to school, she started to buckle under the pressure of the competitive girls in her class. Once again she felt unat-tractive and worthless. Quickly, she fell back into her old pattern of using crystal to cope. She stopped calling Karen because she was embarrassed to tell her that she had relapsed. Part of her also didn't want to hear what Karen would tell her—that she should stop the crystal.

Ana ended up in rehab a second time, and afterward she was referred to an intensive outpatient program to help her make the transition back as she faced the pressures of high school. She is continuing to attend groups and AA meetings. Although she is trying to build a network of friends who are sober and supportive, she finds it extremely difficult in a community of high-school students who like to party with alcohol and drugs. She has already slipped a few times, using crystal on a few occa-sions, but fortunately she keeps going to meetings and groups, and none of the slips have turned into a full-blown relapse yet. After a slip, she is sometimes able to call Karen, and she thinks this may have saved her from another full-blown relapse. Every day Ana reminds herself what she learned during her first rehab: self-esteem is something that can take years to build, and for many it's a lifelong process.

ACUPUNCTURE

IN RECENT YEARS, increasing numbers of people are turning to alternative medicine to treat physical and emotional problems. Because of my work in addiction, I try to teach people to learn new ways to manage emotional discomfort without automatically resorting to pills, though sometimes medication is truly necessary. The addiction-treatment community has long turned to acupuncture as a nonmedication alternative for some of the problems associated with addiction and withdrawal.

One of the earliest pioneers in introducing acupuncture to the addiction-treatment community was Dr. Michael Smith at Lincoln Hospital in the South Bronx of New York City. He opened a drop-in center where people wishing to stop heroin could come for acupuncture to ease their withdrawal symptoms without resorting to medications. Dr. Smith has been criticized by many who say that acupuncture is a scam. However, Dr. Smith also has a large group of supporters: people coming off the streets, almost all of them heavy heroin addicts, many of them homeless. They come in feeling dope-sick and distressed, they line up for acupuncture, and after receiving treatment, they appear remarkably calm and comforted. While the use of acupuncture for medical uses is hotly debated, there is no question that many people receiving treatment at Lincoln Hospital in the South Bronx feel relief.

Most heroin treatment centers that use acupuncture only target needle points in the ear. These points seem to offer heroin addicts the most relief, and because the area is so limited, certification is easy and staff can easily be trained, making the service available to a large number of people. If you are able to see a practitioner who is fully licensed in acupuncture, you can get the additional benefit of treatment with points other than just the ears, balancing the entire system and providing even greater relaxation and relief.

We will discuss acupuncture in more detail in chapter 17, which includes the general principles of how acupuncture works and how you can find a licensed acupuncturist near you.

MEDICATIONS

MEDICATION FOR CRYSTAL addiction remains a new and evolving field as medical science learns more about the biology of the brain and the neurophysiology of addiction. I have already discussed the use of medications for detoxification from acute withdrawal. Here I will discuss several medications under investigation for maintenance treatment of methamphetamine addiction, with the goal of decreasing craving and reducing the number of relapses.

In the past, most of the attention to stimulant addiction, including methamphetamine and cocaine, focused on dopamine agents because stimulants affect dopamine, and this is the major chemical that mediates the brain-reward circuit of addiction. While this pathway is a fundamental part of addiction, there are also many other brain processes, neural pathways, neurotransmitters, and intracellular "secondary messengers" involved. In lay terms, it means that addiction is much more complex than just the dopamine-reward pathway. Unfortunately, nothing as simple as controlling dopamine has turned out to be a magic bullet. To add to the confusion, drugs that *increase* dopamine stimulation and drugs that *block* dopamine stimulation both seem to have beneficial effects on reducing stimulant use in animal studies. Most recently, studies have found that the best effect comes from dopamine partial agonists, which share properties of both the dopamine stimulators and the dopamine blockers.

Other brain structures, such as the striatum, the cingulum, and the cerebral cortex, have been found to have their own important roles in addiction. Neurotransmitters in these areas, such as glutamate, glycine, and **gamma-aminobutyric acid** (**GABA**) are currently under investigation. Dopamine receptors no longer monopolize the spotlight. Researchers are also looking at mu-**opioid** receptors, GABA receptors, N-**methyl-D-aspartic acid** (**NMDA**) receptors, **cannabinoid** (marijuana) receptors, calcium ion channels, DNA gene transcription . . . and the list goes on and on. The more that we discover about the brain, the more enigmatic it becomes.

Because of this early stage in drug trials, it is not possible to make extensive comments on what medications may be helpful in preventing crystal relapses. **At this time, there are no medications approved by the U.S. Food and Drug Administration specifically for the treatment of methamphetamine. Therefore, I can only report on the limited studies of different medications and comment on their theoretical applications for the treatment of crystal addiction. I do not recommend using these medications to treat methamphetamine until studies provide further evidence for their efficacy and safety.**

Topiramate (brand name Topamax) is an antiseizure medication that has been prescribed for pain from nerve damage, migraine headaches, and anxiety. It was later found to reduce alcohol cravings and relapses. Further research showed that it had a similar effect in reducing cocaine relapses. The positive effect on cocaine addiction makes it a good candidate for crystal addiction, because of the similarities between the two drugs. While Topiramate is not addictive, it must be used carefully. It is started at a low dose and gradually increased, because sudden increases in dosage can cause severe mental confusion. Other side effects are decreased appetite and weight loss, countering the hunger and weight gain that often occur when you suddenly stop using crystal. If you are taking topiramate and decide you want to stop, make sure to taper off gradually. Because it is an antiseizure medication, stopping topiramate abruptly can theoretically cause a seizure.

Gabapentin (brand name Neurontin) is also an antiseizure medication. It seems to work very specifically on certain calcium channels in the brain, though its exact mechanism of action remains unknown. Although it functions differently than topiramate, it has been found to have many of the same therapeutic effects, including decreasing anxiety and reducing relapses on cocaine. Trials investigating its effects on methamphetamine addiction are under way.

Acamprosate (brand name Campral) has long been used in Europe to treat alcoholism. It is thought to work by increasing GABA function (helping relaxation) and decreasing glutamate overactivity (decreasing anxiety and brain toxicity), which occurs when alcoholics start to feel strong cravings for alcohol. For people who have stopped drinking, it was believed to prevent relapses by decreasing the intensity of the craving through its effect on blocking overactive glutamate activity. Unfortunately, a recent large-scale study showed that acamprosate was no better than a placebo at decreasing alcohol relapses—while study subjects taking acamprosate showed improvement, it was no better than the subjects taking sugar pills.

Naltrexone (brand name Revia) is an opiate antagonist, blocking the effects of opiates, such as heroin. An intravenous analog called naloxone is used in emergency rooms as an antidote for people who overdose on opiates and stop breathing. Naltrexone, which is taken as a pill, has been used with success in some alcoholics, possibly blocking opiate receptors at reward and pleasure centers that are stimulated by alcohol. With less of a reward, people may not feel as strong a desire to drink. There are other theories about how naltrexone works, such as balancing out the opiate receptors in the brain at its resting state so that the user is happier in general, thus requiring less self-medication to elevate a low mood. Using this theory, naltrexone is now being investigated as a medication for crystal addiction. As a pill, it needs to be taken every day. However, a long-acting injectable form called Vivitrol was recently approved and is soon to be released. Requiring only one injection per month, it offers protection to those in recovery who are very motivated but have sudden moments of weakness, when they stop taking naltrexone pills so that they can drink or use opiates. The most common side effects are stomach upset and rare irritation to the liver. People with hepatitis B or C should be cautious with naltrexone.

Dopamine antagonists are medications that directly block the site of action of crystal: the dopamine receptor. In animal studies, these drugs demonstrate an excellent ability to block the effects of stimulants. However, dopamine receptors are located throughout the entire brain, and in the long term, this class of medication is associated with numerous neurological side effects. It is not likely to be a good candidate for long-term use.

Medications that affect the GABA receptor are generally calming, inhibiting brain cell transmission, including signals that instruct the brain to use more drugs. Theoretically, medications affecting GABA should lower the intensity of drug cravings and decrease the number of relapses. Therefore, there is intensive research on these medications as treatments for stimulant addiction. Clinicians are concerned about the addictive risk of benzodiazepines. However, mild to moderate nonaddictive medications that increase the effect of GABA, such as tiagibine (Gabitril) and baclofen (Kemstro), have shown only modest benefit. Gamma-vinyl GABA (GVG) is the strongest GABA medication available, and a recent study by Dr. Jonathan Brodie found that sixteen of the eighteen people who remained in his study had dramatic improvement in staying off meth. However, GVG has a dangerous risk of patchy blindness, so studies on GVG were halted in this country. Notably, none of the subjects in Brodie's study suffered vision problems, though 15 out of 33 subjects dropped out of the study.

The last medication I will discuss in this chapter is modafinil (Provigil). This drug increases alertness and reduces mental and physical fatigue. To date, studies show that modafinil has an extremely low potential for addiction and that it is effective at reducing and preventing relapses in cocaine addiction. Imaging studies do not show any significant change in the nucleus accumbens, which is usually activated by addictive drugs. For this reason, it is being investigated as a treatment for methamphetamine addiction, and at this time it looks to be one of the most promising treatments currently available. Subjectively, meth addicts in acute withdrawal quickly feel an improvement in their fatigue and the clarity of their thinking.

Modafinil's effect on methamphetamine addiction may be due to its increase in glutamate activity, an important chemical in the brain that deals with learning new behaviors, taking information and weighing options, and then making logical decisions. In addiction, these brain activities affect the ability to resist temptations to relapse. While dopamine and the meso-limbic pathway are responsible for *establishing* the initial addiction, the maintenance phase of addiction is believed to be mediated by glutamate. Glutamate is used to communicate between the brain-reward pathway and the prefrontal cortex, where logical thinking and judgments are carried out. The function of this bridge is important because it determines how well a person can make rational judgments in reaction to strong signals from the brain-reward pathway telling it to use drugs.

In crystal addicts, the baseline level of glutamate activity is low, meaning that the ability of the brain to make proper judgments is impaired, for example, deciding whether to go to a party where all your old meth buddies will likely be getting high. Modafinil seems to increase glutamate in areas where it is too low, and perhaps it improves the ability of addicts to assess their circumstances and make logical judgments.

Crystal users also have an abnormally high spike in glutamate when they see a cue reminding them of crystal. They may experience the spike as a rush of excitement when they hear their dealer's voice or see a picture of a glass pipe that reminds them of times they've smoked. It is possible that modafinil also lowers this spike, which may help addicts to resist sudden urges brought on by the usual triggers that lead to relapse.

These are all theoretical conjectures about modafinil. The exact mechanism in which it works is still unknown. Nevertheless, the early results of current studies of modafinil as a treatment for crystal addicts have been showing promising results. In addition, many physicians, myself included prescribe Provigil in their practices and have seen their meth-addicted patients improve. However, there are a handful of reports of people feeling mild euphoria from modafinil. Two of my patients, both of them with bipolar disorder experienced this. One of them was in recovery from crystal meth. He reported feeling high and energized, with a strong compulsion to take increasing amounts. The second patient was not an addict and did not develop an addiction to the medicine, although he became extremely manic, with racing thoughts, euphoric or easily irritable mood, and so much energy that he needed very little sleep. Because both patients had bipolar disorder, it is still unclear if the patient in recovery from meth addiction was feeling hypomanic and impulsive from taking increasing amounts of modafinil, or if he was having a pure drug relapse. The cautionary point is that, while this medication looks extremely promising as a treatment for crystal addiction, it must be used with caution.

Additional considerations about modafinil are that it is extremely expensive and it interacts with a number of prescription medications, more reasons to be cautious. For example, it increases the metabolism of protease inhibitors (PI) for HIV and particularly affects ritonavir (Norvir). If the PI level becomes too low, it is not able to kill HIV, and strains of the virus that are resistant to the medication can develop and severely worsen the person's health. Dr. Judith Rabkin at Columbia University studied the use of modafinil for fatigue in patients with HIV. In that study, doses were kept to a maximum of 200 mg per day, and there was no effect on the HIV medications in any of the study participants. I recommend caution if you take a PI: be cautious with modafinil, and do not take more than 200 mg per day.

Another significant effect of modafinil is that it can reduce the concentrations of some oral contraceptives in the bloodstream. Women who wish to take modafinil must be aware of this and discuss it with their gynecologists so they can either adjust their oral contraceptive dose or consider other methods of birth control.

As this book goes to press, a new medication called Prometa is being aggressively marketed for the treatment of meth addiction. It is a proprietary combination of three medications that have been in use for a long time, though never for the treatment of meth addiction. The foundation of the treatment appears to rest on the use of flumazenil, a benzodiazepine receptor blocker (i.e., an antidote for medications such as Valium and Xanax). The theory behind this treatment is that flumazenil changes the structure of the GABA receptors in brain cells, which become misshapen from long-term drug use. By changing the shape of the GABA receptor back to its original form, the hope is to decrease cravings for meth. Flumazenil is administered in daily infusions by vein, in conjunction with two other medications taken by mouth.

This medication regimen has been heavily marketed by the corporation holding the proprietary rights to Prometa, through billboard campaigns as well as solicitations of physicians. Aggressive marketing began long before any reliable scientific evidence demonstrated that this treatment was effective, which has caused more worry than optimism in many physicians.

Recently, an open-label study—meaning a study in which all subjects were given the drug—by Dr. Harold Urschel of Research Across America, was completed showing that a remarkable 80 percent of people reported a reduction of meth use. This figure is impressive, but consider the powerful effect of placebos (fake pills) when the person taking the placebo is in the right frame of mind. The subjects in this particular study were likely desperate for an effective treatment after several prior failed medications or therapies. They may have seen billboard advertisements for Prometa making promises of a new drug-free life, and then received a dramatic treatment intervention involving daily intravenous infusions. In other words, the weight of psychological influence in this context is heavy.

While the aggressive marketing tactics for Prometa treatment have made addiction specialists extremely wary, the theory behind the treatment is an interesting one. However, it still needs rigorous scientific testing—which means a study in which half of the subjects are randomly assigned to get a placebo. This type of research is called a double-blind placebo-controlled study, which is considered much more reliable in ascertaining the true efficacy of a treatment. It shows how much of the benefit is due to the drug regimen itself versus the psychological effects of aggressive marketing and taking a dramatic drug treatment regimen.

PEOPLE WITH A "DUAL DIAGNOSIS"—
DEALING WITH ADDICTION AND DEPRESSION, ANXIETY,
OR OTHER PSYCHIATRIC PROBLEMS

"DUAL DIAGNOSIS" is a term used to describe people who have a drug addiction *and* another psychiatric illness, such as depression, anxiety, bipolar disorder, or schizophrenia. In the past, addiction and other psychiatric illnesses were often treated by separate medical specialists, but because each illness affects the other so profoundly, addiction experts strongly advocate treating both illnesses together.

If a person has a dual diagnosis, and one of the two illnesses is left untreated, it is highly likely that *both* conditions will get worse. For example, if meth addiction is not adequately treated, then continued crystal use can trigger depression, bipolar mania, psychosis, obsessive-compulsive thoughts and behaviors, panic attacks, and anxiety. Meth is so powerful that it can render antidepressant medication useless, and people who already suffer from major depression may become even more vulnerable to severe depression and suicide.

Conversely, an untreated psychiatric illness significantly increases the risk of relapsing on drugs. For example, if a person in recovery who has been sober for years becomes severely depressed and suicidal, she may remember the times when she used meth and her mood instantly lifted. In a moment of desperation, she could easily slip, and if she stopped using crystal, she would become more depressed, so she is then locked into a full relapse, unable to stop using crystal. Another example is a man with bipolar mania. In his manic state, his confidence is overinflated and he forgets all he has worked to learn about powerlessness. In addition, mania almost completely eliminates his impulse control—not only is he grossly inappropriate in public, but when the urge to use crystal enters his mind, he may not be able to stop himself. Once he starts using meth, the drug chemically magnifies the manic symptoms, and he spins out of control. With the excessive dopamine released by crystal, he may be at even more risk of a psychotic mania, with hallucinations and delusions. These are only two of many examples that demonstrate how significantly addiction and psychiatric illness can affect each other, and they underscore the importance of treating both illnesses at the same time.

This section will review some basic psychiatric illnesses that commonly occur with addiction and can significantly increase drug relapses, and conversely, these illnesses can be worsened by meth use.

Major depression is a clinical state that includes low mood, among several other symptoms. Depression or low mood can be experienced differently by each individual. Some descriptions include sad, tearful, hopeless, empty, bored, flat, guilty, and worthless. Mood symptoms may be so distressing that the person feels suicidal because life is so painful. Along with the emotional symptoms, there are physical symptoms, including disturbed sleep (increased or decreased), low or restless energy, poor motivation and mental fatigue, changes in appetite (increased or decreased), poor concentration, and a significantly decreased ability to experience pleasure. Depression can follow an upsetting event, but it can also occur for no apparent reason. The medical definition of major depression requires a period of at least 2 weeks with these symptoms, but this time restriction is arbitrary and even 7 to 10 days of these symptoms without any clear reason to feel sad should prompt you to seek psychiatric treatment.

There are numerous antidepressants on the market, each affecting various neurotransmitters and neuropeptides (small proteins that are active in the brain), including dopamine, norepinephrine, and serotonin. These neurotransmitters may help balance mood and decrease the anxiety that may contribute to craving for all addicts, with or without a dual diagnosis. Studies with various antidepressants have had mixed results as far as treating addiction. A recent study of nondepressed meth addicts treated with sertraline (Zoloft) actually showed a dramatic increase in relapses in those who were taking sertraline compared with people taking a placebo. There are many theories to explain this surprising effect: the sertraline may decrease the depression in a crash, so people are more likely to use; the increased transmission in some serotonin fibers may block certain dopamine signals, which could make addicts crave meth even more. There are many more theories, but the answer remains a mystery for now. The major lesson is that the neuropharmacology of addiction is complicated, and people should be wary of taking a friend's psychiatric medications or other supplements to try to protect their brains, when they use drugs. This does not mean that antidepressants increase relapses in everyone—the subjects were nondepressed addicts. When used in appropriate situations, treating clinically depressed people with effective antidepressants can significantly reduce cravings for crystal that can actually be desperate attempts for any relief in their mood, as illustrated in the example at the beginning of this section.

Schizophrenia is a structural imbalance in the brain, with overactive dopamine activity in certain areas and deficient dopamine activity in others. This is one reason schizophrenics are at higher risk for cocaine and crystal addiction—during their first experience with cocaine or crystal, they unknowingly stumble upon a wonder drug that elevates dopamine where it had been low and caused them to feel lifeless, unmotivated, and empty. The reward they experience from crystal may be even more powerful than what nonschizophrenics feel. Unfortunately crystal also increases dopamine activity in areas that are already overactive, making schizo-phrenics even more psychotic, suffering more severe hallucinations and delusions. Treating schizophrenia with the right medication significantly reduces the risk of relapsing. Common medications include haloperidol (Haldol), chlorpromazine (Thorazine), olanzapine (Zyprexa), risperidone (Risperdal), ziprasidone (Geodon), and aripiprazole (Abilify).

Bipolar disorder is brain disorder in which a person experiences alternat-ing periods of depression and overactivation, which can have a euphoric, irritable, or anxious mood accompanied by increased energy, overinflated self-esteem, and difficulty controlling impulses. Even without the extra challenges of mania, the urge to use crystal is powerful and sometime irresistible. When mania is also present, a biological loss of impulse con-trol makes it almost impossible to resist the urge to use crystal. The most extreme forms of bipolar disorder may seem obvious to most people (e.g., the stereotypical comedy representation of two men sharing a jail cell who both believe they are Jesus); however, there are still a surprising number of people who do not believe it is a medical illness, but rather a difficult personality. In its milder forms, when mood swings are not as extreme, it can be harder for people to accept that it is a biological illness. However, studies show that indeed it is. Left untreated, bipolar illness is actually toxic to the brain, leading to destruction of brain cells, which can be seen on imaging studies of the brain. Because of the terrible effect it has on people's lives (25 to 50 percent attempt suicide, and 11 percent suc-ceed in killing themselves), its toxicity to the brain, and its strong impact on addiction and relapsing, it is extremely important to treat it properly with medication. Common treatments include mood stabilizers, such as lithium (Lithobid, Eskalith); valproic acid and valproate (Depakene and Depakote); carbamazepine (Tegretol); oxcarbazepine (Tegretol); lamotrig-ine (Lamictal); as well as the newly developed atypical antipsychotics, such as olanzapine, risperidone, ziprasidone, and aripiprazole.

OTHER IMPORTANT AREAS IN YOUR LIFE TO KEEP YOU CLEAN AND SOBER

Identify Major "Holes" in Your Life That You May Fill with Crystal

Objectives:

- Learn about specific psychiatric conditions such as social anxiety disorder, depression, and attention-deficit/ hyperactivity disorder, which can significantly increase your risk of relapsing if they are left untreated.

- Consider how hard you work, how much you expect from yourself, and whether you have been using crystal as a way to maintain unrealistic expectations.

- Review the concepts of "stress management," "moderation," and "acceptance," which are fundamental to leading a happy life, as well as reducing cravings and relapses.

- Examine your social circle and consider how your friends may help you stay clean or how they may be triggers that pull you back to drugs and using crystal. When forced to end destructive relationships, consider ways of dealing with loneliness and finding a healthier circle of friends.

- Think about how crystal has affected your experiences of sex and consider ways to relearn the pleasure of sober sex.

12

SELF-ESTEEM:
How Much Do You Really Like Yourself?

> Crystal made me confident, even fearless—something alcohol and cocaine could never do. I felt validated through meth-infused sex. A few hours of illusory intimacy were better than days of emptiness. Instead of always being the best little boy in the world, I could run, if only for a few hours at a time, with the fast crowd—the fabulous people.
> —EDDIE YOUNG, quoted in "Living with[out] Crystal Meth,"
> *Positively Aware*, July/August 2005

ONE OF CRYSTAL'S appeals is its ability to elevate self-confidence. While most people would enjoy a boost in confidence, this effect can be particularly compelling for people who have deep-seated feelings of low self-esteem. If the only time you feel good about yourself is when you are high, then meth seems like one of the few things in this world that make life seem worth living. But there are many other reasons that you can feel good about yourself. If you have low self-esteem, ignoring your core beliefs about yourself by masking them with drugs will leave you constantly needing more drugs to protect you from the pain that low self-esteem causes. Semple and colleagues at the University of California at San Diego conducted a study looking at 157 heterosexual male meth users and found that negative self-perceptions strongly predicted the intensity of their meth use and depression. Do you have a distorted, low self-image that puts you at risk for relapsing?

How is *your* self-esteem?

What was your response to that question? Many people instantly respond that they are fine and have no problem with how they see themselves. In fact, the more quickly you respond, "There's no problem," the more likely you actually believe there is something wrong, but you are trying desperately to protect yourself from it and deny it. Remember the famous quote from Shakespeare when Queen Gertrude says to her son, Hamlet, "The lady doth protest too much, methinks." The queen was quite astute, in realizing that the woman in the play she was watching protested so much because she was trying to hide something. (Unfortunately, she was not astute enough to realize that the character in the play she was watching was parodying *her*!) Similarly, all people are capable of responding this way when we try to convince ourselves and others that nothing is wrong. An automatic positive response to the question "How is your self-esteem?" doesn't allow you time even to consider the question with any thought. A quick reply avoids taking the time to examine yourself and possibly seeing something that you don't line. On the other hand, if you took a couple seconds to ponder the question before answering, your response was probably closer to the truth.

Pretending that nothing is wrong seems like a reasonable way to avoid negative feelings—if you say that everything is fine, eventually everything will be fine, right? Indeed, having a positive self-image is healthy, *as long as it is truthful*. However, using superficially positive images that only mask your true feelings is dangerous because the negative thoughts are never addressed, and since they remain unchallenged, they continue to lurk in the back of your mind. Until you take the time to examine those thoughts, you will never address them and make them better.

WHAT IS SELF-ESTEEM?

How do you feel about yourself? As a child, what kind of person did you imagine you would become? Have you become that person of your fantasies? One way to conceptualize self-esteem is to measure how successfully you lived up to your self-expectations. Low self-esteem comes from the disappointment of failing your expectations. Good self-esteem comes from making realistic expectations and feeling the satisfaction of meeting them, or at least being satisfied with why you have not met them yet.

Perhaps you have not wed the prince charming of your childhood dreams because you were busy pursuing a promising but demanding and successful career. Maybe you couldn't finish high school, against your parents' wishes, because they died and your younger brothers and sisters needed you to earn money to feed and shelter them. Perhaps as a child you had fantasies of becoming a professional basketball player, but you grew to be only five and a half feet tall. If childhood fantasies never turned into reality, is it because you truly are a failure, or is this just where life ended up taking you, while you deal with life in the best way you can?

WHERE DO EXPECTATIONS COME FROM?

THOUGH MANY OF us try to be open-minded, as hard as we try not to make assumptions, to accept people just as they are, and to accept our own situations—our lot in life—it is a natural human process to form expectations. We have expectations about everything—ourselves, other people, common occurrences, such as the fact that summer should bring with it warmer weather. In many instances, they are helpful: when we are expected to attain certain level of performance at work; it helps keep us motivated and productive. The problem arises when expectations are unrealistic—if they are impossible to meet, then they are guaranteed to cause disappointment. There are three ways to deal with this: (1) change our expectations to make them more realistic; (2) feel intense disappointment but continue to have the same unrealistic expectations, which likely leads to further disappointment; or (3) take extreme measures to meet the expectations. Option 1, trying to keep your perspective in line with reality, is the healthiest. Options 2 and 3 are dangerous because they are stressful and unrealistic, and can lead to drug relapses. For example, if you hold on to the same expectation, which you repeatedly fail to meet, you may treat the disappointment with drugs, rather than change the source, which is the distorted expectation. In the third example, if you try to take extreme measures to meet the unrealistic expectation, such as trying to meet an impossible deadline, then you may resort to drugs like crystal to accomplish this. Only the first option, making your expectations more realistic, will help you in a healthy and long-lasting way.

Many of our expectations—of ourselves, of others, and of situations—are based on similar experiences from our recent past that help us to assess whatever is happening at the moment. Here's an example: "There are hundreds of people on the subway platform. I haven't seen it this crowded here since there was a major breakdown in the tracks. I bet the subway system is having trouble, and I don't expect I'll make it to my appointment on time." However, we also hold expectations of ourselves or others without such an obvious basis—for example, they could result from distant, buried experiences from long ago, childhood fantasies of how we *wished* things to be, traumatizing childhood disappointments that our minds try to protect us from ever experiencing again. Expectations based on distant experiences and memories are extremely powerful because, in most cases, we are not entirely aware of why we have them. Perhaps this is because they are rooted in experiences stored so deeply in our minds that they feel like "unquestionable realities," and perhaps they are difficult to question because we aren't aware of the reasons to challenge. Even when the expectations are unrealistic and cause unhappiness, we often simply accept them. Consider for example, a wealthy businessman who is never satisfied with his company and is constantly driven to make more money. Another case is a best-selling writer who, despite excellent reviews and record-breaking book sales, has a burning need to produce something better. If you speak with her, you can see her creative enthusiasm, but you can feel that something else is pushing her, that there is something she is trying to prove to herself. These are not unusual examples. In fact, they are quite common illustrations of how much of our behavior is influenced by these mysterious self-expectations.

Most of our expectations, both conscious and unconscious, are shaped by our earliest life experiences. Like sponges, babies and small children absorb everything from their environment. During this early stage of human development, babies and children begin to form a rudimentary understanding of good versus bad, and the actions and words of the people around them help them figure out what falls into each category. Along with a general concept of right and wrong, children have both internal fantasies—their own innate desires—and external messages—encouragements, demands, and explicit expectations that others tell them—of what they *should* be, as well as what they should *never* be.

For example, a mother tells her little boy, "Your father and your grandfather worked so hard to build the family business, and when you're an adult, you'll take over the company! We'll be so proud of you! You know, that company is what this family is built on, and it's very important for you to keep it going when you're older and it's your turn." Another message that used to be commonly heard, both at home and in some school home economic classes, was, "If you want to be a happy woman, you have to be able to cook well for your husband, so make sure you learn how to cook!" More subtle messages that children pick up are statements as simple as: "Don't do that! What will others think?" The majority of messages children hear are attached to strong emotions, as well as judgments of right and wrong: the little boy feels pressure to take over the family business because any desire to do anything else would disappoint his beloved parents, even if he were not interested in the company at all; the girl hears a message that her happiness is determined by marrying a man and then doing whatever it takes to please him—a compelling message for any human being who wants to be happy. Even as we grow older, develop our own interests, and have rational ideas of what would best make us happy, those childhood messages, so heavily weighted with our earliest beliefs about what determines happiness or sadness, quietly linger and affect how we feel about ourselves and what we expect ourselves to be and to do.

The most significant role models for children are usually their parents. To some degree, we all inherit some of our parents' expectations, whether we agree with them or not. A common experience is for a boy to say, "When I grow up, I'll never act like Dad!" Then, one day in his adult years, he hears himself scolding his own children and says, "Did I just say that? I'm acting just like my father!"

Even if children angrily disagree with their parents, they unknowingly internalize many of their parents' expectations. Despite the rebellious attitude of many teenagers who are trying to develop a sense of independence, *all* humans have some innate desire to please their parents, This is true even if they are only aware of disagreeing with their parents and feeling anger toward them.

What did your parents expect of you? Did they expect you to go to college and become a wealthy businessman? Did they expect you to get married, imagining themselves happily surrounded by the grandchildren they expected you to have? These parental wishes may become yardsticks that you unconsciously use to measure our own success or failure, as well as your feelings of satisfaction or disappointment in whatever you do.

For gay men, internalized expectations of parents often become a tremendous source of unconscious disappointment and self-loathing. All children receive messages about sexuality constantly, through words from their parents, friends, and teachers; from television shows and movies, from watching people on the street; and even from simple magazine advertisements and commercials. Many homophobic people say to gay people, "Don't flaunt your sexuality in front of the whole world!" The reality is that every television show that includes heterosexual people mentioning a spouse, child, or potential love interest, a jewelry commercial that shows a diamond engagement ring, or a travel brochure with a picture of a man and woman holding hands on the beach—all of these are "flaunting" heterosexuality. Children are constantly bombarded by these messages that tell them, "Life is supposed to culminate in a heterosexual relationship, marriage, and children, and the ultimate goal in life is to continue the family name." Even the most "out and proud" gay man may struggle with a deeply hidden, disapproving "yardstick" that leaves him feeling that in the end he still does not measure up.

Understanding your unconscious expectations is a long process, best done with the help of an experienced therapist. However, the following two exercises provide ways to start your self-exploration, and to see what buried and hidden beliefs may still be affecting your behavior and your self-esteem today.

EXERCISE 12-1 PARENTAL EXPECTATIONS

PARENTS are the people with whom babies and small children have the most social contact. Because children have a natural desire to please their parents, their expectations are particularly compelling. Ask yourself the following questions about your parent's attitudes. Can you see any of them in how you judge yourself?

- As a child, do you remember if your parents felt proud of you? Disappointed? Satisfied? Ashamed? Frustrated? A combination of different feelings? Do you remember any *predominant* feeling?

- Were you ever confused about how your parents felt about you? Did they ever give you confusing messages, such as, "Congratulations for winning the silver medal! Too bad you couldn't get the gold." Did you feel they were beaming with pride? Did you think they were disappointed? How did you feel about your parents at that moment? How did you feel about yourself?

- How far did your parents expect you to go in school?

- Did your parents push you to get good grades? How hard? If they did not push, did they care about grades or how well you did? Did they focus on other things in your life that they thought were more important? Did they not believe you were capable of doing well? Did you feel that your parents generally weren't concerned about you?

- How did your parents react to your school performance? Were they proud? Were they indifferent? Were they worried at times but encouraging? Were they angry? Do you remember this ever affecting how you felt about your intelligence or your own abilities?

- Did your parents help you whenever you needed assistance, or did they encourage you to be "strong" and to do things for yourself? How did this make you feel? Abandoned or neglected? Stronger and more capable? Weak, like a failure?

- Did your parents ever ask you about who you were dating? Were they uninterested? Were they intrusive, asking a lot of questions or giving a lot of advice to point you in "the right direction"? Did they ever disapprove or seem disappointed? Were they open and supportive? How did that affect your attitude toward your own romantic and sexual feelings?

- Did your parents ever tell you what they wanted you to become when you grew up?

- What did your parents imagine your life would be like when you reached age thirty?

- Did your parents ever say they wanted grandchildren? As a child, did you ever imagine yourself as an adult with children? If you answered yes, why do you think that as a child, you were already

thinking about having a baby? What was the motivation behind
that fantasy?
- When your parents imagined their own later years in life, how did
you fit into their picture?

EXERCISE 12-2   SOCIETY'S EXPECTATIONS

IN addition to the influence of parents, children continue to learn social
norms as they grow up, absorbing general society's ideas as if they were
axiomatic truths. As adults, we are taught to think rationally, and most believe that logic governs our behavior more than the older ideas we picked
up during childhood. However, consider the phenomenon of the dreaded
high school reunion. The purpose of reunions is enjoyment, but many, if not
most, people attend them feeling excitement that is mixed with feelings of
anxiety and dread. Reunions are unusual occasions when old, uncomfortable beliefs about former classmates' judgments and expectations come
back to the surface. Many feel a pressure to prove their success, that they
were able to meet or exceed their classmates' expectations. Why does a
regular job feel acceptable at other times, but at a reunion it might feel
like a source of shame? The influence of other people's expectations may
have seemed dead and buried, but at a reunion, you realize that they have
always stayed with you, and only now are they so apparent.

What were the expectations that you learned from your peers when you
were growing up? Answer these questions to clarify what they might be.

- What did most of the other kids like to do in elementary school?
What games did they play? In junior high and high school, what
were most people interested in? Sports? Hanging out at the mall?
Playing video games? Dating? Going to parties and drinking alcohol or doing drugs?
- What did you like to do in high school—were they the same things
as everyone else, or were they different? If they were the same,
how did you feel about that? If they were different, how did that

make you feel? Did the differences have any effect on how you saw yourself? Did you feel smarter, dumber, prettier, uglier, less popular, or an outcast? Did you wish you could fit in better or did your differences make you determined to be the opposite, so off-beat that you could feel cool in your own way and avoid the worry about being like everyone else?

- How did other kids in school treat you? Were you a popular student with a large following? Did this make you feel confident and free or did you feel pressure to behave a certain way because you were afraid of losing people's respect? Were you somewhere in the middle, with a group of nice friends but wanting to be with the more popular kids, striving to look and act like them and hoping to one day be one of them? Were you mistreated by your classmates, rejected for being different and not allowed to be part of the group? How did your classmates' treatment make you feel about yourself?

- Did most of your classmates graduate from high school? Was it rare that kids in your school attended college? Did most of your classmates go to college or graduate school? How far did you go in school, and how did this make you feel about yourself?

- What kinds of jobs and lives did your classmates imagine for themselves? Did they want to stay in their hometown and get any job that would pay the bills? Did they want to move away, get a particular job, or want to make a tremendous amount of money? Did they plan to marry or have children? When you were in school together, how did your own hopes and dreams compare to your classmates'? Were they the same? If they were different, how did that make you feel? Did you talk to your classmates about how different your plans were? If not, what thoughts and feelings held you back?

- What are your classmates doing now? Are they working? What kinds of jobs do they have? Are they single, married, or divorced? Are they gay or straight? Did they have children?

- What was the "macho" expectation for guys in high school? What was the "feminine" expectation for the girls?

- In your class, how did you fit in?

After completing exercises 12-1 and 12-2, consider the expectations of your parents and classmates and the many ways in which those expectations were communicated to you. How closely does your life compare to the expectations of your parents and classmates? Going through the exercise, along with other people's expectations, think about your reactions to them—how they made you feel about them and yourself. Did you feel content and satisfied, or did you feel different? Did you want to fit in more or to please your parents better? Did you try to free yourself of those expectations and take a completely different path? These two exercises are not in-depth explorations of your personality, but they help you to understand that some of your self-expectations are from people, places, and times outside of your immediate awareness. Knowing this, you can search beyond the surface appearance of your motivations to look at what they really are. Regardless of your job success, number of sexual conquests, accumulated wealth, or whatever you have achieved, according to the deeper self-expectations which you may still hold, are you a success or a disappointment? Unconscious expectations can be harsh, irrational, and unrealistic. Therefore, it is important to identify any hidden expectations you hold yourself to and understand where the expectations come from and the reasoning behind them. Knowing these things, you can assess whether they are appropriate or whether they need to be revised.

Ultimately, self-acceptance and self-satisfaction determine happiness. The less you accept yourself, the unhappier you are. Drugs offer a temporary way to address disappointments because they artificially alter the way you feel about yourself. "Downers," such as alcohol or heroin, make people care less or feel numb to disappointment. Stimulants, such as crystal and cocaine, can pump up feelings of self-worth, allowing users a temporary sense of confidence, power, and attractiveness. For some, using may be the only time when they genuinely feel good about themselves. Unfortunately, these positive feelings are artificial and last only as long as the drug high because there is no fundamental change in the cause of low self-esteem. Many people simply try more crystal to feel better again, digging themselves deeper and deeper into addiction. The better way to address bad feelings, as well as to avoid relapsing, is to develop a stronger, more positive sense of self.

WHAT CAN I DO TO IMPROVE MY SELF-ESTEEM?

SELF-ESTEEM IS a deep-seated character trait. It took your entire life to evolve into what it is now. That is why quick-fix remedies, such as repeating the mantra "I love myself!" or simply telling yourself, "Everything's fine!" do not really work. They may give you a temporary boost, and remind you that you *should* love yourself and feel worthwhile, but they do little to actually change how you see yourself. If you never address those nagging, hidden self-expectations, they will continue to haunt you and make you feel inadequate.

Psychotherapy can make profound and lasting improvements in your self-esteem, but the process can be long, and ongoing therapy may not be a realistic option for you. There are also cognitive strategies that take a different approach, which is still effective for many and can also have long-lasting effects.

The following exercise works on the belief that disappointment results from not fulfilling your self expectations. If your expectations are unrealistic, then you are bound for disappointment. The exercise, divided into five parts, clarifies what your expectations are, compares them to your real life situation, and examines why they do or do not match. Adjust your expectations so they are realistic, and then you can assess how well you've met them. If you still haven't met these revised expectations, at least these expectations are logically constructed, and you can think of rational ways to meet your goals.

EXERCISE 12-3a EXPECTATIONS

LIST expectations you *currently* have or *used* to have about your own life in the following areas. Include rational expectations, but also include any childhood fantasies you may have had (e.g., I wanted to be an astronaut; I used to dream about becoming Miss America; I want to be the next Donald Trump; I wanted to be the first black, female president of the United States).

Education

_____

_____

Appearance

_____

_____

Occupation

_____

_____

Income

_____

_____

Relationships

_____

_____

Other miscellaneous areas

_____

_____

EXERCISE 12-3b REALITY

HOW does your reality compare to the expectations in exercise 12-3a? What have you achieved in the following areas? Did you meet, fail, or surpass those expectations?

Education

_____

_____

Appearance

_____

_____

Occupation

_____

_____

Income

_____

_____

Friendships

_____

_____

Romantic relationships

_____

_____

Other miscellaneous areas

_____

_____

EXERCISE 12-3c EXPLAIN THE DIFFERENCE

IF certain aspects of your life did not turn out as you had expected, what are the reasons? Here are some possible explanations: Did you have poor grades in school because you never actually gave it a good *try*? Were you afraid that if you tried and failed, then this would prove that you were undeniably stupid? Did you try a particular job but, even with your best efforts, you *couldn't* do it? Did other job opportunities come up in life, which you chose instead because they seemed *more promising*? Did your interests *change* over time, and you decided to pursue something more interesting while your parents' expectations remained the same? Were there *unavoidable reasons* for not being able to fulfill the expectations? For example, if telling your family and classmates you were gay caused violent reactions and rejection, did that affect your performance in school or make you rebel against your family and peers and pursue the *opposite* of their expectations? Did angry or abusive parents kick you out of the house and take away the financial support that would have helped you finish school? Did you wish to be a beautiful, blonde-haired woman with blue eyes, but being in an ethnic minority and having black hair and brown eyes, were you never able to see yourself as pretty? Did you think you wanted to be a doctor because your parents and all your brothers and sisters were physicians, but biology bored you and the sight of blood made you faint?

In each category, try to explain why any of your original expectations did not match how your life actually turned out.

Education

_____

_____

_____

_____

Appearance

_____

Occupation

Income

Friendships

Romantic relationships

Other miscellaneous areas

EXERCISE 12-3d REVISE YOUR EXPECTATIONS

CONSIDER the reasons you gave in exercise 12-3c for not meeting your expectations. Are they justifiable? Are there areas that you think you should still work on? Consider your life experiences; your knowledge about yourself, your interests, and your abilities; the challenges you face each day; and the other unavoidable circumstances of your life. With these in mind, go through the same categories and write *realistic* expectations for yourself in each.

Education

_____

_____

Appearance

_____

_____

Occupation

_____

_____

_____

Income

_____

_____

Relationships

_____

_____

Other miscellaneous areas

_____

_____

EXERCISE 12-3e HOW TO WORK ON AREAS THAT REALLY
NEED IMPROVEMENT

THERE may be some expectations that you find still make sense, and though you haven't met them, you wish you could., With a logical understanding of your expectations, your abilities, and your challenges, what *specific* things can you do to meet those expectations? If you always wanted to get a college degree, can you return to school or take night classes while working? Are there ways that you can advance in your career? Have you fully investigated job opportunities, talked with a career counselor, or contacted a headhunter? If you are dissatisfied with your appearance, are there ways that you can improve the body you have in a healthy way? In summary, are there *realistic* ways to reach the goals you have set for yourself? If you have unmet expectations that are achievable, then making a concrete plan and seeing that they are attainable will give you a sense of hopefulness and control, and you will already be on your way toward higher self-esteem.

Education

_____

_____

Appearance

_____

_____

Occupation

_____

_____

_____

Income

_____

_____

Relationships

_____

_____

Other miscellaneous areas

_____

_____

This five-part exercise encourages you to think about self-expectations in a systematic, organized way; confronts you with difficult self-perceptions; and helps correct "cognitive distortions," which are unrealistic thoughts that you held on to, silently affecting the way you experience yourself and the world around you.

Digging up old and buried expectations and addressing them directly, rather than hiding from them, will help you improve your self-esteem. If you find that your self-esteem is extremely low, it may take a long time to raise, but this exercise can serve as a springboard for more intensive work in psychotherapy. Working on yourself over the long term doesn't sound as easy or as attractive as drugs, but it will be far more rewarding as you begin to feel truly happy with yourself. Repeat this exercise from time to time to see if your answers to any of these questions have changed. You may be surprised at how your answers change as your self-esteem rises.

Reaching a Better Understanding of Himself BRIAN'S STORY

In addition to attending CMA meetings, Brian started to see a psychiatrist who explored his self-esteem issues and deep-seated notions of low self-worth. He had thought he was comfortable with being gay—he had come out to his family and all his friends in his midtwenties, and outside of work, he considered himself "comfortable" with his sexuality. However, Brian started to see how he quietly harbored feelings of shame about his sexual orientation, guilt for disappointing his parents, and anger and hatred toward himself. Gradually he understood that he was angry and disappointed at his inability to be what his parents wanted, so he tried to show them, as well as himself, that he was still worthwhile by becoming a successful attorney. "Was that the fire that kept me fueled to sit through all those boring law-school lectures I hated so much?" he asked himself. He realized that no amount of work was going to address his parents' view of homosexuality—if that were to change, he'd have to tackle it in a different way that would address his real dissatisfaction.

Brian also found that some of his anger mimicked the hatred toward gays that he witnessed growing up. He had always thought that joking with his gay friends about effeminate men and casually using works such as "queen," "queer," "fag," and "Mary," were ways of accepting his sexual orientation. But they were also ways that he held on to the homophobia he had learned as a child. Sometimes his anger became an intense, irrational rage toward himself that he hadn't completely understood: at times he thought to himself, "How could I let myself be such a pathetic loser?" despite his hard work, successful career, and good looks. Suddenly he recalled a time in high school when he felt such self-loathing and despair because of being gay that he contemplated different ways to kill himself.

Accepting himself as a gay man was not as simple as admitting that he was gay, and Brian found that he had not been as comfortable with his sexual orientation as he had thought. All of the negative feelings and self-expectations he inherited from others contradicted his natural attraction and desire to be with men. This made sex and relationships terribly confusing because despite knowing that he wanted to be with men, his pleasure was always tainted by unclear bad feelings.

Brian gradually worked on improving these parts of his self-esteem, and he was able to feel better about himself—not in a temporary drug-induced way, but in a long-lasting, fundamental understanding of himself. He didn't need crystal to help him with that aspect of his life anymore. Brian still had urges to use and had a few slips. But he stuck with his treatment program and created a network of sober gay professionals he could connect with in ways other than drugs and circuit parties. He felt connected, accepted, and validated, both as a gay man and as a human being. At the time of this writing, it has been two years and five months since Brian has used crystal.

13

SOCIAL ANXIETY:
When It's Difficult to Feel Comfortable
Around Other People

SOME PEOPLE USE crystal to help them manage social situations because of its positive effect on their confidence. Quiet people who are usually wallflowers at parties may start to feel talkative, engaging, attractive, powerful, and desirable. Having always felt left out, they finally see themselves able to participate in the world, at least when they are using meth.

Social anxiety is quite common. Most frequently, it is simple shyness, feeling timid, and slow to warm up to others. It is usually associated with some anxious belief that others will see the person in a bad way. Shy people are quiet with strangers, but usually they can still function well in life. More extreme social anxiety is considered a disorder called **social phobia** or **social anxiety disorder**. When shyness reaches the level of social phobia, the fear of embarrassment becomes so intense that it is difficult or impossible to face people and get through day-to-day life. These people withdraw or rarely go out of the house because their anxiety is so disabling. This doesn't mean they don't *want* to be around others—on the contrary, they want desperately to interact with people. However, their fear imprisons them in their loneliness, and they feel miserable. While meeting all of the criteria for social phobia may be extreme, a great number of people suffer from a lesser degree of social anxiety or shyness that still significantly worsens their quality of life.

The DSM-IV criteria for social phobia are listed in table 13-1:

TABLE 13-1

DSM-IV Criteria for Social Phobia

SOCIAL PHOBIA

A. A marked and persistent fear of one or more social and performance situations in which the person is exposed to unfamiliar people or to possible scrutiny by others. The individual fears that he or she will act in a way (or show anxiety symptoms) that will be humiliating or embarrassing. Note: In children, there must be evidence of the capacity for age-appropriate social relationships with familiar people and the anxiety must occur in peer settings, not just in interactions with adults.

B. Exposure to the feared social situation almost invariably provokes anxiety, which may take the form of a situationally bound or predisposed Panic Attack. Note: In children, the anxiety may be expressed by crying, tantrums, freezing, or shrinking from social situations with unfamiliar people.

C. The person recognizes that the fear is excessive or unreasonable. Note: In children, this feature may be absent.

D. The feared social or performance situations are avoided or else are endured with intense anxiety or distress.

E. The avoidance, anxious anticipation, or distress in the feared social or performance situation(s) interferes significantly with the person's normal routine, occupational (academic) functioning, or social activities or relationships, or there is marked distress about having the phobia.

F. In individuals under age 18 years, the duration is at least 6 months.

G. The fear or avoidance is not due to the direct physiological effects of a substance (e.g., a drug of abuse, a medication) or a general medical condition and is not better accounted for by another mental disorder (e.g., Panic Disorder With or Without Agoraphobia, Separation Anxiety Disorder, Body Dysmorphic Disorder, a Pervasive Developmental Disorder, or Schizoid Personality Disorder).

H. If a general medical condition or another mental disorder is present, the fear in Criterion A is unrelated to it, e.g., the fear is not of Stuttering, trembling in Parkinson's disease, or exhibiting abnormal eating behavior in Anorexia Nervosa or Bulimia Nervosa

Reprinted with permission from the *Diagnostic and Statistical Manual of Mental Disorders*, Fourth Edition, Text Revision (Copyright 2000). American Psychiatric Association.

Whether you meet full criteria for social phobia or have a significant degree of social anxiety, you may be using crystal as a way to cope—you've found something that makes you feel and function better when you use it. But the effect is only temporary. It doesn't change the person you are or your fundamental fears of what people think of you. You know from experience that once the high disappears, you will return to the same shy person you were before. You may feel even worse during the crash after using. It eventually becomes a trap, because you see that you can function well socially and feel acceptable, but the only way to keep this up is to keep using.

One way to address problems with socializing that is healthier and longer-lasting than using crystal is to examine your self-esteem (see chapter 12) and change the negative core feelings that you have about yourself. Most of your shyness is probably based on false beliefs about yourself and your fear of how other people see you. An anxious reaction to these beliefs turns it into a self-fulfilling prophecy. You think you appear awkward, you become increasingly nervous, and when forced to speak, you may be so overwhelmed by anxiety that your voice trembles, you become red or covered in sweat, or you blurt out something strange which you would never have said under normal circumstances—you are too distracted by your anxiety to think clearly and say what you mean. You aren't a fool, but if you allow it, your fear will convince you that you are.

Consider an Olympic gymnast who has to mentally focus on her takeoff, her body position at every moment of her routine, and her landing. Distraction by the smallest thing can throw off her performance, and if she is distracted by overwhelming anxiety, her performance will be terrible.

Think of the boxers who stare into the television camera or at their opponents and growl, saying that they are going to destroy the other fighter. Both fighters say the same thing, though it is impossible that they will both win. Some of this is bravado and showmanship—they need the fans, the ratings, and the ticket sales. But much of this is to prepare themselves mentally. They need to elevate their self-esteem, and they cannot allow themselves to be distracted by fear. In the same way, if they can scare their opponents and can fill them with self-doubt, the opponent will not perform as well.

Self-perception has a tremendous effect on a person's performance, even if that person is truly skilled. If you use crystal to artificially ease your social discomfort, you will never address how you actually see yourself, and without the drugs, your negative self-perception will always be there, making you uncomfortable around other people. On the other hand, if you directly address your fears and reactions, then you give your true strengths a chance to shine. This becomes a self-fulfilling prophecy, as well. The more you see yourself socially effective without drugs, the more you believe in yourself, and the more your confidence shows, and the better you function in social situations. And this no drug—this is a real change in you.

WHAT CAN YOU DO TO LOWER SOCIAL ANXIETY?

Improve Your Self-Esteem

The first step in lowering social anxiety is to examine your real thoughts and beliefs about yourself. How do you see yourself? Where do those thoughts and beliefs come from? Are they based in reality? See chapter 12 for a detailed discussion on this topic and exercises on how to improve your self-esteem.

Practice Your Social Skills

One of the most basic and most effective treatments for social anxiety is **cognitive-behavioral therapy** (**CBT**). CBT involves intensive work and it is extremely challenging. Like training for an Olympic competition, CBT is a long road of pushing yourself through uncomfortable exercises, with small, incremental gains at any one point. However, the overall gain is tremendous and long-lasting.

The cognitive part of "cognitive-behavioral therapy" examines the way you think about yourself. Is your view distorted for some reason? Gather some data. Ask other people how they see you, especially people who know you well. Strangers or superficial acquaintances may be more familiar with the shy you, but people who know you well, such as your family and friends, know what you are like when you are not anxious. Exercises 13-1 through 13-3 help you to find any cognitive distortions and correct them.

EXERCISE 13-1 HOW DO YOU PERCEIVE YOURSELF
IN SOCIAL SITUATIONS?

EVEN if you feel fine about yourself when you are alone, your comfort and confidence may evaporate when other people are around you. Answer the following questions about how you *imagine* you appear in social settings, such as parties or office meetings. Even if your fantasies seem irrational, try to be as honest as possible about your thoughts and fears (e.g., "Everyone is looking at me" or "I seem so boring and nobody cares what I have to say"). Use these questions to help you consider different ways you may view yourself, and feel free to include any areas not listed.

How do you imagine other people see you?

_____

_____

_____

How do you imagine you sound when you talk in a group? Do you seem intelligent? Do you seem nervous? Do you seem as if you know what you are talking about? Do you seem stupid or silly?

_____

_____

_____

Do you ever say anything interesting? Are you concerned that people are bored or annoyed when you speak?

_____

_____

_____

Do you think that anyone has ever been attracted to you? Why or why not?

_____

_____

_____

_____

What are things that other people may like about you?

_____

_____

_____

_____

Do you think there are any other positive things that people think about you when you talk with them?

_____

_____

_____

_____

Do you think there are any other negative things that people think about you when you talk with them?

_____

_____

_____

_____

EXERCISE 13-2   WHAT ARE MY REAL STRENGTHS
AND WEAKNESSES AND HOW DO OTHER
PEOPLE ACTUALLY SEE ME?

ASK the following questions of family members and friends *with whom you are comfortable and familiar.* These are the same questions as in exercise 13-1, but they examine an outsider's perspective.

How do I look to you?

How do I sound when I talk to you? Do I seem nervous? Do I seem as if I know what I am talking about? Do I seem stupid or silly?

Do I *ever* say anything interesting?

Do you know if anyone has ever been attracted to me?

What are things that you like about me?

Is there anything else positive that you notice when we are together?

Is there anything negative that you notice when we are together?

EXERCISE 13-3 IDENTIFYING COGNITIVE DISTORTIONS

WERE there any differences between what you imagined about yourself in exercise 13-1 and what your family and friends thought in exercise 13-2? This will help you to understand how different your fears can be from reality. These differences are called cognitive distortions, and the distortions need to be corrected. Simply knowing that the fears are irrational is not enough to make them go away. However, with a list of cognitive distortions to work on, you have a focus and can address your fears constructively.

For each of the differences that you found in exercises 13-1 and 13-2, write the following statement:

I fear that when I am around people, others will see me as _____

_____.

However, the reality is that people have seen me as _____

_____.

EXERCISE 13-4 CORRECTING COGNITIVE DISTORTIONS—
A BEHAVIORAL APPROACH

ONCE you know the false assumptions that you make, use them in this technique of behavior therapy.*

Pick a specific fear identified in your list of cognitive distortions in exercise 13-3, e.g., "When I approach strangers and introduce myself, they think that I sound stupid." Start with one of your less challenging fears. Your task will be to do this specific act *at least ten times* in one day. Repeat this exercise daily for five days—this means repeating the act a total of at least fifty times. Make the task simple and quick. For example, if you are in a party, go up to ten different people you don't know, casually introduce yourself, and say, "Hello, my name is Pat Smith. Nice to meet you." Keep the interaction brief and say something positive and simple, such as, "This is a great party, isn't it?" Have a standard exit line, such as "Oh, no! Please excuse me, I need to find my friend Jamie. It was a pleasure meeting you." and move on. Remember, in *this* exercise, your only goal is to say hello, not to make new friends. Limit your interactions, as you are concentrating on overcoming your anxiety from one specific behavior—approaching strangers and saying hello. If you linger and try to interact further, other sources of anxiety may arise, and the benefit of the exercise is lost.

This technique is called **exposure with response prevention (ERP)**. The more you expose yourself to a fearful situation, the less sensitive you become to it. After each exposure, you will find that your level of anxiety decreases. Optimally, you should do these exposures in quick succession for your mind and body to learn from the experiences. If you do this exercise only once every two weeks, every day that you do not do the exercise, you reexperience your old fearful reaction, and you relearn your fear response. The next time you do the exercise two weeks later, it may feel like you are starting from scratch.

---

*Behavior therapy is an effective method of changing emotional responses by repeatedly exposing a person to something to elicit a specific response. In the case of anxiety, behavior therapy repeatedly exposes a person to something he or she fears and trains the person's body to stop having the biological responses of anxiety.

Expect that the first few times you do this exercise, your anxiety will be high, and indeed you may appear a little awkward to others. Nonetheless, continue to repeat the exercise. Remind yourself that even if you feel stupid at first, it is not because you *are* stupid—it is because you don't feel confident. The more times you repeat the behavior, the clearer it will become that even if you blunder, nothing terrible actually happens. Intellectually you learn this through observing yourself. Biologically, your body is unable to keep up a sustained state of anxiety, so if done in rapid succession, your body's anxiety response will decrease. Both mentally and physically, you become desensitized to your fear.

The first few times you do this exercise, concentrate solely on completing the task. After a few repetitions, if your anxiety has decreased somewhat, you will feel less overwhelmed each time you expose yourself to the situation. At that point, you can observe yourself and the people around you, and you are better able to compare your cognitive distortions to what actually happens when you do the exercise. In our example of approaching people to say hello, take note of the following:

1. What was the other person's response to you? Was the response what you had imagined?
2. How do you think you seemed to the other person?
3. How uncomfortable or anxious was the situation for you?

As you continue the exercise, continue to gather data about your cognitive assumptions and distortions.

This is a labor-intensive exercise, much more that doing a bump of crystal. However, it pays off tremendously because it is effective and the improvement endures—and there is no crash afterward! If anything, some people feel a high from the confidence and rush of accomplishment. In addition, this exercise teaches you a way to deal with anxiety of any type, demonstrating that you can overcome it yourself. If you are persistent with this exercise, you will gradually start to incorporate this method of repeated exposure and desensitization into other aspects of your life without even noticing it, and you may develop your own automatic ERP techniques to handle anxiety.

Medications

If behavioral techniques are not possible because you are so anxious that you are unable to try exercise 13-4, then your social anxiety may be extreme enough to require medication. The most effective medications for this type of anxiety are **selective serotonin-reuptake inhibitors** (**SSRIs**). Serotonin is involved in many functions of the brain, including cognition (thinking and memory), mood, impulsivity, and different aspects of motivation. Studies of baboons, which have strict hierarchies, show that the more dominant baboons have higher brain levels of serotonin, while serotonin levels in brains of those at the bottom of the chain were the lowest. It is not clear if serotonin causes dominance or, conversely, if social success increases brain levels of serotonin. Regardless, numerous studies show the relationship between serotonin and social behavior, and serotonin-related medications have been investigated and used successfully for people with social anxiety. Methylenedioxymethamphetamine (MDMA), commonly known as Ecstasy, is an extremely powerful serotonin agent, which induces intense feelings of social bonding and closeness. Likely this is one of its greatest appeals for marginalized or nonmainstream teens who often go to rave parties, as well as gay men at discos and circuit parties. Both groups struggle with experiences of social rejection, and the social bonding effect of Ecstasy can feel tremendously healing. Unfortunately, Ecstasy is also toxic to the brain, and the effect on social connections is short-lived.

SSRIs affect serotonin in a gentler nontoxic manner, and they have been found to be extremely effective at decreasing social anxiety. Ask a psychiatrist to see if this medication is appropriate for you. Each brand of SSRI has its own unique side-effect profile, so there may be a process of trial-and-error to determine which is best for you. Also, initial side effects take some time to resolve, while the therapeutic effects begin after several weeks—this is the price for taking a medication that is effective but extremely safe and nonaddictive. Knowing this beforehand may decrease the frustration of finding the right medication. But the wait is worth it. *Psychiatric medications should always be taken under the direction and supervision of a physician familiar with them.*

Another major class of medication that helps with social anxiety is **serotonin-norepinephrine reuptake inhibitors** (**SNRIs**). They increase levels of both serotonin and norepinephrine, and they may be an effective alternative to SSRIs, if you can't find one that works well for you.

Taking psychiatric medications for social anxiety does not necessarily mean you will need to take them for the rest of your life. If you work closely with a therapist, then medications may be only a temporary part of your treatment. Optimally, you should work with a therapist to address social anxiety, whether or not you take meds. However, if you do take meds, a therapist will monitor your feelings closely during treatment as you do exercises such as those in this chapter to work on the core psychological beliefs behind your anxiety. Watch yourself interacting with others effectively and store these images in your mind, internalizing observations of yourself as a socially competent person.

If you decide to stop medication, taper off in small increments. Unlike with crystal, cocaine, and Ecstasy, you may not notice the loss of effect for several weeks or months with each decrease in dose. If social anxiety returns, the small decrease in your dose should allow only a small increase in anxiety, and this less intense anxiety will be easier to address with behavioral exercises, such as exercise 13-4. As you become less anxious again, try another small decrease in medication, and repeat the behavioral exercises. Eventually you may find that you do not require medications at all. Medications should always be gradually tapered, to prevent any possible withdrawal discomfort that occasionally occurs. Symptoms can range from mild body aches, dizziness, and fatigue, to moodiness or spontaneous crying. *Again, medications should always be taken under the supervision of an experienced physician.*

An important class of medications to mention is the benzodiazepines, including medications such as Valium, Xanax, Klonopin, and Ativan. These medications treat anxiety quickly. They were discussed as one of several ways to help with the extreme distress some people feel during a crash. However, benzodiazepines are addictive, particularly if you already have an addiction. In the crystal detox protocol outlined in chapter 9, they are used with extreme caution and given only in a small, limited amount. If you use them regularly, they can increase your risk of relapsing onto crystal, even though they have a completely different effect than meth. An important rule of thumb is to *avoid taking any potentially addictive drug*. Remind yourself that you are taking medications, practicing cognitive-behavioral exercises, and treating anxiety in order to treat your crystal addiction. You do not want to make your addiction worse, and you certainly don't want to pick up a new one.

A BRIEF NOTE ABOUT PSYCHODYNAMIC PSYCHOTHERAPY

Psychodynamic psychotherapy is based on the principles of psycho-analysis, the school of psychotherapy most popularly associated with Sigmund Freud. Encouraging the patient to think by free association, psychodynamic therapy delves deeply into your personality, uncovering what may lie in the unconscious (unaware) mind that influences your behavior. It focuses on three aspects at understanding you: (1) your present life; (2) the distant past from childhood, which forms the template for how people experience the world as adults; and (3) the relationship between the patient and the therapist as a model of how the patient experiences and interacts with people in general. The fundamental concept is that problems arise when things that your mind wants to do differ from what your conscience thinks is the morally right thing to do. This "conflict" creates an inner crisis, so the unconscious tries to find a compromise, which often results in problematic behavior that we can't seem to stop.

Deep exploration of these conflicts takes years of intense self-examination. For some, it can be an extremely rewarding way to understand one's own character and to see the hidden conflicts that may cause certain problems, such as low self-esteem despite making great achievements, feeling trapped in a dissatisfying career, or difficulty having successful relationships. There is a gradual change in people's underlying character, as fears, insecurities, and conflicts are addressed, and, through a process of working through issues, character changes in a lasting way. The following is a very simple example of unconscious conflict that may be resolved in therapy:

Christina **is a 30-year** old woman frustrated in her search for the right man to marry. She wants a husband who is kind, honest, and treats her well—not too much to ask for, she thinks. However, for some unknown reason, whenever a man she dates turns out to be truly honest and caring, she discovers something else about his personality that is so annoying that she cannot tolerate him anymore, and she starts looking elsewhere for love.

In psychodynamic therapy, Christina discusses how she had been "Daddy's little girl," with cheerful memories until she was seven, when her father suddenly died. She was too young at the time to understand what had actually happened. When Christine turned twelve, her mother told her that her father had been hit by a drunk driver. When she heard the explanation, her reaction was anger at the driver who killed her father. However, when she was seven, all she could think of was her intense sadness and confusion when the person she loved most in the world was suddenly gone. In therapy she also recalled feeling tremendous rage at her father for leaving her.

In the therapy, Christina began to see her own fear of getting married because falling in love would put her at risk of being abandoned and devastated again. The connection became clearer when she was talking about her anger, and her thoughts associated to her last boyfriend and her intense anger at him for occasionally coming home late from work.

In the therapy, as she felt more connected with the therapist and opened herself up in sessions, she occasionally noted anxiety that her therapist would leave her or sudden feelings of intense annoyance at him for things she had seen him do many times before without any emotional reaction. Using this as an example, Christina was able to work through her fears and rage with her therapist and develop a sense of trust and stability in relationships. She noticed that she started feeling less angry at her boyfriend of the time. The quality of her relationships improved, and at age thirty-four, she met a man she eventually married.

Psychodynamic psychotherapy is such a rich field that it is impossible to discuss it in detail in this book. In addition, it is mentioned here as a type of therapy for later in recovery because I discourage exploratory therapy during the initial stages of sobriety, until addicts have stronger relapse prevention skills and are able to handle the emotional stress that usually arises as you uncover deep and unconscious feelings. However, later in recovery, when sobriety skills are strong, psychodynamic psychotherapy can be extremely helpful to understand and improve the self, as well as address deeper character issues that may be the root of some addiction problems.

14

DEPRESSION:

When Nothing Feels Good—
Is This the Way Life Is Supposed to Feel?

CRYSTAL HAS AN amazing ability to elevate mood. People who are depressed can feel almost instant relief when they use it. One of the ways it works so quickly is by releasing massive amounts of dopamine, one of the neurotransmitters that improves mood and thinking. When the drug effects wear off, the brain has much less dopamine than before, and the depression can become even worse than it had been before using crystal.

Some people who have been medically diagnosed with major depression take antidepressant medications. These medicines increase the availability of such neurotransmitters as dopamine, serotonin, and norepinephrine by preventing their removal (termed "reuptake") from the spaces between brain cells. While they do not increase *production* of these neurotransmitters, they help the brain to maximize the usage of what is already in the brain in order to maintain stable mood. Crystal, on the other hand, releases so much dopamine that it depletes the brain of its dopamine reserves. In addition, it prevents brain cells from producing more dopamine, so it is not able to replenish its depleted supply. With little dopamine left, there is nothing for antidepressant medications to work on, thus, they may lose much of their effect or become entirely useless.

If you suffer from an underlying depression, a chronically low mood puts you at high risk for relapsing because you are searching for anything to make it feel better. If you have tried crystal, your brain already knows that doing just a little can snap you out of a painful depression, even if only for a brief time, and even if the price is worse emotional pain afterward. When depression is severe, you may be desperate for any kind of relief, no matter what the cost. To avoid the risk of relapsing, you need to know if you have an underlying depression. If you do, you must treat it aggressively, both to lead a better life and to reduce the risk of relapsing on crystal.

WHAT IS DEPRESSION?

"Depression" is such a commonly used word in the English language that its exact meaning is unclear. In the medical field, we use the term **major depression** to refer to a specific biological state of the brain.

Depression, in the broadest sense, means low mood. The stereotype of a depressed person is someone who is always sad or crying. However, "depressed mood" can be experienced in many different ways that are not as easy to recognize. Some people experience depression as unhappiness without actually feeling sad or tearful. Depressed people may also describe their moods as hopeless, helpless, guilty, heavy, empty, bored, flat, joyless, dark, irritable, unmotivated, low, distressed, or simply "bad." All humans feel these emotions at certain times. When terrible events occur in life, it is *appropriate* to feel unhappy. Depression, however, is different from a bad mood, because the negative feelings are not appropriate; (1) they may occur even when there is no identifiable cause; and (2) depressed people become stuck in their low mood—they feel depressed most of the time, and no matter how hard they try, they cannot shake the feeling, even long after most people would have recovered from a sad event. Whatever the cause, depressed people have an inability to feel happy or experience pleasure, and they long to end the emotional pain and to feel normal again. Depression can last several weeks to months, and sometimes it can last for years.

In addition to low mood, major depression has several other symptoms— it is a physiological state of the brain and body. In addition to mood, some physical symptoms include changes in sleep, appetite, and energy; poor concentration; low motivation; mental fatigue, a decreased threshold for bodily pain, and a decreased ability to experience pleasure. Depression is not simply a bad attitude or a weak character; it is a medical condition, which may require medical treatment, such as medications, in addition to therapy.

If you are depressed and do not address it properly, then recollections of the euphoria of crystal can make the desire to use again irresistible, seeming like the only way to find relief.

WHAT IS "MAJOR DEPRESSION"?

PHYSICIANS USE A definition of depression using strictly defined criteria. The broad range of symptoms reflects how multiple bodily functions other than mood are involved, underscoring the biological nature of depression. Technically biological depression is called **major depressive disorder**. Table 14-1 lists the criteria for a **major depressive episode** as it is defined in the DSM-IV:

TABLE 14-1

DSM-IV Criteria for Major Depressive Episode

MAJOR DEPRESSIVE EPISODE

A. Five (or more) of the following symptoms have been present during the same 2-week period and represent a change from previous functioning; at least one of the symptoms is either (1) depressed mood or (2) loss of interest or pleasure.

Note: Do note include symptoms that are clearly due to a general medical condition, or mood-incongruent delusions or hallucinations.

1. Depressed mood most of the day, nearly every day, as indicated by either subjective report (e.g., feels sad or empty) or observation made by others (e.g., appears tearful). Note: In children and adolescents, can be irritable mood.

2. Markedly diminished interest or pleasure in all, or almost all, activities most of the day, nearly every day (as indicated by either subjective account or observation made by others)

3. Significant weight loss when not dieting or weight gain (e.g., a change of more

than 5% of body weight in a month), or decrease or increase in appetite nearly every day. Note: In children, consider failure to make expected weight gains.

4. Insomnia (difficulty falling asleep or staying asleep) or hypersomnia (sleeping too much) nearly every day.

5. Psychomotor agitation or retardation nearly every day (observable by others, not merely subjective feelings of restlessness or being slowed down). [For example, pacing, rocking, hand-wringing]

6. Fatigue or loss of energy nearly every day.

7. Feelings of worthlessness or excessive or inappropriate guilt (which may be delusional) nearly every day (not merely self-reproach or guilt about being sick).

8. Diminished ability to think or concentrate, or indecisiveness, nearly every day (either by subjective account or as observed by others)

9. Recurrent thoughts of death (not just fear of dying), recurrent suicidal ideation without a specific plan, or a suicide attempt or a specific plan for committing suicide

B. The symptoms do not meet criteria for a Mixed Episode.

C. The symptoms cause clinically significant distress or impairment in social, occupational, or other important areas of functioning.

D. The symptoms are not due to the direct physiological effects of a substance (e.g., a drug of abuse, a medication) or a general medical condition (e.g., hypothyroidism).

E. The symptoms are not better accounted for by Bereavement, i.e., after the loss of a loved one, the symptoms persist for longer than 2 months or are characterized by marked functional impairment, morbid preoccupation with worthlessness, suicidal ideation, psychotic symptoms, or psychomotor retardation.

Excerpted from the Diagnostic and Statistical anual of Mental Disorders, Fourth Edition

Dysthymia is a milder form of depression that is not as severe as major depression. The degree of low mood may not be as severe, and there may not be as may not be as many physical symptoms. However, the time course of dysthymia is much longer, lasting for at least two years and often much longer. Because dysthymia is not as dramatic and it is so longstanding, it is often overlooked. After feeling mild unhappiness for such a long time, people with dysthymia begin to believe that this emotional state is how life is supposed to feel. Table 14-2 lists the DSM-IV criteria for dysthymia.

TABLE 14-2

DSM-IV Definition of Dysthymia

DYSTHYMIA

A. Depressed mood for most of the day, for more days than not, as indicated either by subjective account or observation by others, for at least 2 years. Note: In children and adolescents, mood can be irritable and duration must be at least 1 year.

B. When depressed, the patient has 2 or more of the following:

   1. Poor appetite or overeating

   2. Insomnia or sleeping too much

   3. Low energy or fatigue

   4. Low self-esteem

   5. Poor concentration or difficulty making decisions

   6. Feelings of hopelessness

C. During this 2-year period, the person has never been without the symptoms in Criteria A and B for more than 2 months at a time.

D. No Major Depressive Episode has been present during the first 2 years of the disturbance; i.e., the disturbance is not better accounted for by chronic Major Depressive Disorder, possibly in partial remission.

E. There has never been a Manic Episode, a Mixed Episode, or a Hypomanic Episode, and criteria have never been met for Cyclothymic Disorder

F. The disturbance does not occur exclusively during the course of a chronic Psychotic Disorder, such as Schizophrenia, or Delusional Disorder.

G. The symptoms are not due to the direct physiological effects of a substance (e.g., a drug of abuse, a medication) or a general medical condition (e.g., hypothyroidism).

H. The symptoms cause clinically significant distress or impairment in social, occupational, or other important areas of functioning.

Excerpted from the Diagnostic and Statistical Manual of Mental Disorders, Fourth Edition

Both major depression and dysthymia can be extremely disabling. People with these disorders feel miserable, and they have a diminished ability to experience pleasure, even when everything in life is going well. Major depression is fairly common, with a lifetime risk of 10 to 25 percent among women and 5 to 12 percent among men. Dysthymia is less frequently noted, with a reported lifetime prevalence of only 6 percent. However, because the symptoms are more subtle and many people never seek treatment, the *actual* prevalence is likely much higher.

Depression of any type can increase your risk of relapsing on crystal because the drug is a quick fix that can make that depression disappear instantly. In the long run, however, it actually worsens depression. If a person is biologically depressed when using, then the crash can be even worse. If a person has had major depression in the past but is not depressed when he or she uses crystal, the crash can trigger another major depressive episode, and what starts out as just a crash can turn into an intense, long-lasting depression. If you have a history of depression, using meth is playing with fire—it may seem exciting, but it is dangerous and can leave you burned. It is particularly risky for you, and you should avoid it altogether.

The best way to treat depression is with psychotherapy and appropriate medication when necessary. These are nonaddictive, long-lasting ways to improve your mood. If you have any signs of depression, it is important to see someone, whether it is your family doctor, a psychiatrist, or a therapist, to have this formally evaluated. As long as you are depressed, you have a greater chance of relapsing on crystal.

15

WORK:

When You Need to Keep Your
Job Performance and Productivity High

DO YOU FIND that it is difficult for you to accomplish all the responsibilities of your job? Are you usually too tired to finish your work, or is the job is so big that it exhausts you? This chicken-or-the-egg question is very important because often, when people are not able to complete a job, their bosses, and even they themselves, assume that it is their own inadequacy. However, it is important to consider whether the *job itself* is really the problem. Almost all jobs have periods of increased or decreased intensity—deadlines, due dates, seasonal fluctuations in businesses and markets. However, if you find that your job *always* seems difficult to keep up with, then this is a problem. If you need crystal or some other stimulant to be able to perform your normal workload, is that really the right job for you?

Many people have used meth to help themselves accomplish more work: cramming for exams, writing last minute papers, or completing work projects by their deadlines. But what starts as a one-time work aid for a special project can become a constant requirement to be able to function at school or work. Some may quickly become addicted to the drug itself, and their constant use keeps them working at an inhuman pace. For most, however, it is a gradual process, in which, having seen what they were able to do on meth, they begin to impose higher expectations on themselves. They accomplish more and more projects with meth, eventually they become used to operating in high gear with little sleep and long work hours. If crystal-fueled productivity becomes your new standard for work performance, it can be an impossible standard to maintain without crystal. At first, this technique may seem to work Over time, the same amount of meth becomes less effective, and you need to use more to accomplish the same job. As you increase your use, you also start suffering more of meth's toxic effects, such as anxiety, distractibility, paranoia, irritability, and disorganization, which, ironically, make your work suffer as well. But by that point, your addiction is so strong that it is difficult or impossible to stop using. The crystal that once made you a star at work may now lose you your job.

If you are trying to recover from crystal addiction, keep your workload reasonable. If this is not possible, the job is not safe for you, and you need to consider another job. This is important advice for all people, regardless of whether they are addicts. Moderation in everything you do, recreational or work related, is important in maintaining a healthy balance of productivity and rest that will prevent you from burning out. "Work hard and play hard" has become an American ideal—strive to be as productive as possible, and reward yourself equally with pleasure. If you put out superhuman productivity, you expect superhuman compensation in return, and a drug high can seem like the perfect reward. This lifestyle is a setup for relapse.

Take a moment to step out of your work, where the momentum of the job can make you assume that the work expectations are reasonable. Independent of your current job situation, what are you striving for in your professional life? What do you really want out of your job? What does your boss expect of you, and what do you expect of yourself? Set high standards for yourself, but keep them realistic and healthy. If they are too high, you set yourself up for disappointment. Some people scramble desperately to avoid disappointment by any means, such as using crystal or other stimulants to help them meet unrealistic goals. Before relapsing, take the time to consider carefully what you really want out of life, and then decide whether your job is able to help you achieve the life you want. You are human, and you have limits—it is all right if you can't do everything in life. Accepting your limitations is far better than trying to meet an unrealistic expectation with drugs.

If you believe your work goals are realistic, is something else preventing you from reaching those goals at work? Depression, social anxiety disorder, attention-deficit/hyperactivity disorder, problems at home, the job itself, or personality issues concerning a coworker or supervisor? If you identify the real obstacle, then you can tackle it, instead of using a temporary solution like crystal, which can eventually turn from a solution into its own problem.

A frequently underrecognized factor that can impair work performance is attention-deficit/hyperactivity disorder (ADHD), and because of the effect of stimulants on this disorder, many people with ADHD have accidentally turned to meth for help. Read the next chapter if you suspect this may be an obstacle for you in your daily life or at work.

16

ATTENTION-DEFICIT/HYPERACTIVITY DISORDER:
You're Not Lazy or Depressed,
So Why Do You Still Have Trouble
Getting Things Done?

IF YOU ARE having difficulty focusing on your work but the work itself does not seem like it should be a monumental task, **attention-deficit/hyperactivity disorder** (**ADHD**) may be what is preventing you from focusing and accomplishing things that should be easy for someone with your intelligence. ADHD is a medical condition that causes difficulty in initiating certain tasks, mentally focusing on uninteresting material, and filtering out distracting stimulation, such as noise or activity around you. Some people with ADHD experience restlessness and severe discomfort when trying to sit still. There are several medications that dramatically improve mental function. The most well-known medications for ADD and ADHD are stimulants, such as methylphenidate (Ritalin) and amphetamines (Adderall), which are similar to crystal, except that they have a much milder effect.

Because crystal is a powerful stimulant, its effect on people with ADHD can be so dramatic that the reason for its appeal is obvious. But the drug is so powerful that it goes beyond treating the ADHD and causes addiction.

Beyond a certain point, it no longer improves concentration but worsens mental function.

One must be extremely careful in making a diagnosis of ADHD. The diagnosis has been overused to explain people's difficulty focusing. This may be the result of several factors: (1) The name of the illness itself is misleading—"attention deficit disorder" implies that any person with problems with attention has this disorder. The reality is that many things can impair attention, including anxiety, depression, bipolar disorder, schizophrenia, dementia, brain injury, prescription and over-the-counter medications, drug and alcohol use or withdrawal, physical pain, and countless medical illnesses; (2) In small doses, stimulants improve concentration in almost all people, misleading people to believe that a positive experience after taking a stimulant definitely means that they have ADHD; and (3) American culture emphasizes the quick fix and the easy solution. The idea that taking a pill could instantly improve one's mental function is extremely appealing to many. Similarly, physicians pressured to see more patients in less time may feel eager to find the simplest and quickest solution to help their patients. The result of all of these factors has been the unintentional overprescription of stimulants. However, when people with ADHD are correctly diagnosed, the appropriate treatment can dramatically improve their lives.

The DSM-IV divides attention-deficit/hyperactivity disorder into three subgroups: a predominantly inattentive type, a predominantly hyperactive-impulsive type, and a combined type. The formal criteria are listed in table 16-1.

TABLE 16-1

DSM-IV Criteria for Attention-Deficit/ Hyperactivity Disorder

ATTENTION-DEFICIT/HYPERACTIVITY DISORDER

A. Either (1) or (2):

1. Six (or more) of the following symptoms of inattention have persisted for at least 6 months to a degree that is maladaptive and inconsistent with developmental level (i.e., that is more than would be expected compared to a child's same-age peers):

Inattention

a. often fails to give close attention to details or makes careless mistakes in schoolwork, work, or other activities
b. often has difficulty sustaining attention in tasks or play activities
c. often does not seem to listen when spoken to directly
d. often does not follow through on instructions and fails to finish schoolwork, chores, or duties in the workplace (not due to oppositional behavior or failure to understand instructions)
e. often has difficulty organizing tasks and activities
f. often avoids, dislikes, or is reluctant to engage in tasks that require sustained mental effort (such as schoolwork or homework)
g. often loses things necessary for tasks or activities (e.g., toys, school assignments, pencils, books, or tools)
h. is often easily distracted by extraneous stimuli
i. is often forgetful in daily activities

2. Six (or more) of the following symptoms of hyperactivity-impulsivity have persisted for at least 6 months to a degree that is maladaptive and inconsistent with developmental level [i.e., that is more than would be expected compared to a child's same-age peers]:

Hyperactivity

a. Often fidgets with hands or feet or squirms in seat
b. Often leaves seat in classroom or in other situations in which remaining seated is expected
c. Often runs about or climbs excessively in situations in which it is inappropriate (in adolescents or adults, may be limited to subjective feelings of restlessness)
d. Often has difficulty playing or engaging in leisure activities quietly
e. Is often "on the go" or often acts as if "driven by a motor"
f. Often talks excessively

Impulsivity

a. Often blurts out answers before questions have been completed
b. Often has difficulty awaiting turn
c. Often interrupts or intrudes on others (e.g., butts into conversations or games)
d. Some hyperactive-impulsive or inattentive symptoms that cause impairment were present before age 7 years.
e. Some impairment from the symptoms is present in two or more settings (e.g., at school [or work] and at home).
f. There must be clear evidence of clinically significant impairment in social, academic, or occupational functioning.
g. The symptoms do not occur exclusively during the course of a pervasive developmental disorder, schizophrenia, or other psychotic disorder and are not better accounted for by another mental disorder (e.g., mood disorder, anxiety disorder, dissociative disorder, or a personality disorder).

Excerpted from the Diagnostic and Statistical Manual of Mental Disorders, Fourth Edition

If you think that you might have ADHD, here are some important points to consider:

- **ADHD is a lifelong biological condition.** Unlike other possible reasons for impaired attention, ADHD is notable from early childhood, and it is likely active even at birth. The DSM criteria states that symptoms must be present before age seven because this is when most children start school and are put into a structured environment, so this is one of the first times that children are forced to focus for any sustained period of time. If attention problems started *later* in life, ADHD is not the reason you have difficulty concentrating. If attention problems are episodic and vary with your mood or events that occur in your life, then it is extremely unlikely that you have ADHD.

- **A positive response to stimulants does not necessarily mean that you have ADHD.** Many people have tried a friend's ADHD medication, such as Ritalin, Adderall, or Metadate, and they found that they were able to focus better. But this response alone does not mean that they have ADHD. Almost everyone focuses better to some degree with stimulants, though as you increase the dose of the stimulant, anxiety and excitement also increase with use, and concentration may actually become more difficult. Conversely, most people with ADHD actually find that stimulants slow down their thinking and give them a feeling of quiet and calm.

If you suspect that you have ADHD, you should see a psychiatrist or psychologist and have a formal evaluation. If indeed you have ADHD, then you should seek appropriate treatment. Fortunately, there are now many nonaddictive, nonstimulant treatments for ADHD, which can improve your quality of life, enhance your mental functioning, and decrease your risk of relapsing onto crystal. In addition, there are many nonmedication behavioral strategies that can help you to keep organized and optimize your focus. If you have an addiction to crystal, then using stimulants to treat ADHD is *not* a good option for you because it mimics the activity of meth too closely and puts you at serious risk for relapse.

17

LIFE IS A BALANCING ACT:
Stress Management

A CARDINAL RULE in relapse prevention, for crystal addiction, other chemical dependencies, and as a general rule for life, is to minimize or manage stress. Anxiety and stress are natural feelings in life. Mother Nature gave our bodies the ability to feel stress to motivate us to do things, whether we are running from a predator for survival or working in hard in school to get good grades. Cortisol, one of the hormones involved in stress, illustrates how stress functions in our lives. The adrenal glands secrete the hormone cortisol in response to physical or emotional stress. A person with inadequate cortisol function, also called adrenal deficiency, generally suffers from fatigue, dizziness, and weight loss, among several other symptoms. However, in the setting of a severe stress, such as a bacterial infection, the inability of the body to mount a normal stress response by increasing cortisol production can lead to dangerously low blood pressure, shock, and possibly death. Clearly, stress has its place in life.

However, all good things must be kept in moderation, or they cause problems. Feeling overloaded from stress can also be extremely problematic. With regard to crystal addiction, too much stress that is not managed properly can lead to a crystal relapse. In addition to giving you energy that can help you do more work, meth can offer an escape from the drudgery of your job to a state of artificial happiness, it can distract you away from unpleasant feelings, it can boost a low mood caused by chronic frustration, overwork, and fatigue, or it can feel like a well-deserved reward for your hard labor. When you are vulnerable from too much stress, there are so many attractive fruits hanging from the forbidden tree of Eden that it can be extremely difficult to resist the temptation to pick one for a bite of sweet, delicious relief.

Medical studies looking at the physiological responses to stress, anxiety, and depression have consistently shown that high levels of stress or depression adversely affects almost every organ system. Some examples of the broad range of negative effects include: exacerbation of high blood pressure, worsening heart health, decreased survival rates in depressed people who have had previous heart attacks, slower wound healing, and impaired function of immune cells, which are needed to fight infection— this last example is of particular importance to people with HIV, who need to optimize their immune function, which is already compromised by the virus. Brain imaging studies give visual proof of the physically toxic effects of anxiety and depression, showing destruction of brain cells in certain areas, compared to people who were treated for these conditions. Most of us can recall some experience in which stress affected our bodies: intense physical or mental stress may have caused some women to miss their menstrual period; both men and women may have more outbreaks of herpes or acne during particularly difficult times. Excessive stress is dangerous in many ways because of the increased the risk of relapsing onto crystal and its myriad negative impacts throughout the human body.

There are two different ways to approach managing stress: (1) preventing it from overaccumulating, and (2) finding ways to counter it when it is unavoidable—an example would be having an effective outlet to relieve stress, such as regular exercise. A good stress management plan should address stress from both directions.

PREVENTING STRESS FROM ACCUMULATING TOO MUCH

IF YOU ARE feeling stressed, it is important to look find the source. Is it your job? Your relationship? Family conflict? Whatever the cause, you need to identify it. Sometimes the source is obvious, but sometimes it is not so clear. For example, someone may be stressed because of working long hours at an overly demanding job. Others may be working long hours at work, but they stay at the office late because the real stress is something outside the office, such as family conflict, low self-esteem and loneliness outside of the workplace, problems coming to terms with one's sexual orientation, and so on. In those cases, working long hours may be an attempt to escape the real source of anxiety, which may be conscious or outside of the person's awareness. The less obvious cases may require some in-depth detective work, and a therapist may be a valuable resource in helping your investigation.

Identifying the source of the stress is an important first step. Only then can you address it. What is the cause of the stressful situation? For example, do you routinely work late hours because you will lose your job if you do not maintain an unrealistic workload? Or do you linger at the office because you are reluctant to go home, where you dread the angry arguments you regularly have with your spouse?

After pinpointing the cause of stress, how can you effectively address it? If home is usually a battleground where you usually argue with your partner, how can you communicate more effectively? Have you considered couples' counseling? If there a conflict with a coworker, can you ask a supervisor to intervene and mediate the problem so that your daily interactions are less unpleasant? If your job is too demanding, can you discuss this with your boss and try to work out a more realistic plan for how to accomplish the work—perhaps setting a more practical time frame, hiring an assistant or additional employees to work on a project with you, or restructuring the project.? If you have been silent about your frustration at this job but nothing has improved, and talking with your boss is not helpful, should you consider working somewhere else?

Just the initial act of creating a plan of action to deal with a problem can be therapeutic because it gives a framework to your stress, which may have been somewhat vague and unclear; it keeps your attention focused on reaching a better state, and making a list of strategies to address the problem may give you some sense of taking control. If you hide from the problem, for example by mentally escaping through drugs or physically avoiding the stressful place, the problem will continue, and growing feelings of powerlessness and hopelessness simply compound the stress.

Regaining control by addressing the problem is an important part of lowering stress.

If you already know what things in general make you unhappy, you are in a great position to prevent future stress by avoiding those situations. If you know that you do not work well in a large corporate environment, or that you cannot tolerate jobs that normally require ten- to twelve-hour workdays, then you should avoid those types of jobs. If you know that interactions with certain people or family members make you feel anxious, annoyed, or angry, even after countless sincere efforts to address the conflict, then figure out different ways to interact with them that will limit your contact to whatever is necessary, but no more. Clearly understanding your own likes, dislikes, and vulnerabilities will not only help you get out of stressful situations, but it can also help you avoid getting into them in the first place.

FINDING AN OUTLET FOR YOUR STRESS

CERTAIN THINGS IN life are unpleasant but unavoidable. In those cases, it is important to have effective ways of coping with your negative feelings. If you think of stress as pent-up energy that accumulates inside you, it is intuitive that periodically some of the energy needs to be released to reduce the pressure we feel inside and allow us to feel calm. Consider the anxious discomfort of an extremely full bladder and the feeling of relief and calm after urinating and releasing the built-up pressure. Some people find that exercise is helpful, such as running, biking, weight training, or other sports. Exercise literally expends energy that has built up inside, and makes you tired, which can also help you to rest and sleep better. It also increases your body's levels of dopamine, norepinephrine, and serotonin, as well as releasing endorphins, your body's own natural opiates. These effects explain why exercise has some antidepressant and antianxiety effects similar to many psychiatric medications. These findings as well as multiple other studies show that exercise improves mood.

Some people find that physical activities that explicitly release aggression, such as boxing or martial arts, help them decrease tension. In addition to the benefits of exercise discussed above, these particular sports also allow you to redirect feelings of frustration and anger in a safe way. For example, hitting a punching bag can symbolically represent your boss who, while angry about something unrelated to you, yelled at you last week.

Complaining about it right then might have cost you your job, but if you never address your feelings, you will carry around the anger, which will add to other stresses that accumulate over time. Fighting sports can help you redirect your unexpressed frustrations in a meaningful but safe way. They can help you feel more in control because in addition to expending energy, practicing a "fighting art" can counter the feelings of powerlessness from your situation.

Be cautious. If hitting a punching bag while imagining your boss's face on it does not bring you relief but makes you ruminate on your problems even longer, then this is *not* a helpful activity. In this case, aggressive fighting sports only perpetuate your anger and prevent you from letting go of your negative feelings. In that case, find a different activity to relieve stress before you build up so much anger that you find yourself in trouble.

RELAXATION

IN ADDITION TO expending pent-up energy, another strategy to reduce stress is relaxation. If you think of exercise as a way of "pushing out" negative energy, think of relaxation as a gentle way of "releasing" those feelings, letting them go. Letting go is another fundamental concept in relapse prevention and twelve-step philosophy. For successful recovery from addiction, you need to let go of trying to have total control by admitting that you have an addiction problem that you cannot manage alone; let go of crystal from your life, and let go of tension and stress before they overwhelm you.

People have developed countless ways to relax, from chanting ancient Buddhist mantras to taking a nice, hot bath—with so many possibilities, you need to find an activity that fits you well. For example, some people find meditating by chanting in a group to be extremely soothing and relaxing. Some may feel it is not their style and makes them feel awkward and uncomfortable—rather than help you feel better, it could increase your stress. Some suggestions for easy strategies to clear your head when you need to calm down include strolling through the neighborhood, taking a leisurely drive (*not speeding*), sitting on a park bench watching the squirrels play, relaxing in front of your favorite TV show, or watching a movie at the local theater. Here are some tips for getting the most out of these and other similar activities:

1. *Do the activity a leisurely pace, and give yourself enough time to do it.* If you only give yourself 30 minutes to take a break and go to the park, but it takes 10 minutes to get there and 10 minutes to get back, then the whole experience becomes a hurried task—just another burdensome task on your list of things to do. Either give yourself more time or pick a place to relax that is closer.

2. *Keep your focus on the relaxation activity.* If you are walking or driving, look at the road, at the scenery around you. Be more aware of your surroundings and enjoy the break from your day—take in the view. Do not just go through the motions of walking or driving while your mind continues to churn as you worry about the stressful deadline you have to meet or replay in your head the angry fight that you just had with your spouse. By focusing on your immediate surroundings, you redirect your attention to the present, and away from your anxieties that lie in the past or the future. Take a mental vacation, and use the time to clear your head and let go of your unpleasant feelings.

3. *Do not place any expectations on yourself while doing your relaxation activities.* While you are walking, you don't need to reach a certain goal in a certain amount of time. As you look at the scenery around you, you don't have to feel the joy of resplendent nature—if you expect your walk in the park will be like Walt Disney's *Bambi*, you'll likely feel disappointed and annoyed that you wasted your time. While the ultimate goal is to make you feel better, the activity itself doesn't really matter. Promise yourself not to set any expectations, and do not worry about feeling better during the relaxation activity itself. It is all right not to feel anything. If you set up *another* expectation, your effort to relax becomes just another test to see if you will pass or fail. The mere fact that you are engaging in the activity means you have already met your goal, so feel satisfied with that and focus on the activity.

4. *Empty your mind of anything outside your activity and let the other things go.* Focus on each step of what you are doing, where your body is, what is around you. Observe your surroundings and just take them in. Diverse schools of thought from widely different philosophies all seem to converge on this point. Western psychology describes it as refocusing your attention away from stress. Zen Buddhism

teaches the concept of *mushin* (no mind). Yoga masters emphasize the importance of centering your mind on the present, to bring unity to the mind, body and spirit—not allowing you to distract yourself with worries about the past and the future.

In addition to the quick fixes listed above, the following are some examples of activities, each with different highly evolved philosophies, all specifically meant to help you to relax. These are only cursory descriptions, but if any of them pique your interest, I encourage you to find out more and give them a try. You may be surprised that you like something completely new. If not, move on to something else. You should have at least one or two activities that you can turn to for relaxation. Whatever activities you choose, make sure they feel right for you.

Yoga

Yoga is an ancient spiritual discipline originally developed in the Indian subcontinent five thousand years ago. The basic text of Yoga philosophy, the *Yoga Sutras of Patanjali* were written in the second century B.C., though this formalized Yoga philosophy was a systemization of a number of older spiritual traditions that had existed thousands of years earlier. Yoga strives to attain a higher state of consciousness and freedom from the cycle ignorance, worldly suffering, and rebirth. Modern yoga has evolved into several branches, each emphasizing different methods of achieving the common goal of enlightenment. For example, Hatha yoga uses a combination of gentle postures and breathing techniques to purify the mind, body, and spirit, while *Pranayama* breathing exercises try to clear the channels in the body that carry the universal life force, called *prana*.

Yoga meditation styles are so varied that it is impossible to generalize the experience. For example, certain schools emphasize gentle techniques, focusing on breathing and balance; others can be extremely intense and physically challenging, with intricate, difficult poses; Bikram yoga is a series of intricate poses practiced in extreme heat, which induces euphoria and profound inner calm in some but which is intolerable to others.

From a medical and psychiatric perspective, many aspects of yoga make sense in a Western, scientific sense. The various breathing techniques and body positions change blood flow to the brain and to the other parts of the body in ways that are unusual in ordinary sedentary life. The breathing techniques help with relaxation because of the amount of oxygen and carbon dioxide that your body accumulates or breathes off. Certain breathing techniques stimulate the **vagus nerve**, which runs through the chest and lower neck. Through various neural connections, the vagus nerve connects to several parts of the brain, including certain fibers in the thalamus that decrease activity in the frontal cortex and lower anxiety; the hypothalamus, improving alertness and attention, and producing feelings of satisfaction and pleasure; and the limbic system and forebrain-reward systems, inducing feelings of pleasure and bonding.

The effects of vagus nerve stimulation have been well documented in medical literature, and a device called a vagus nerve stimulator (VNS) was developed to treat depression that did not respond to conventional medications. The VNS is implanted in a procedure similar to implanting cardiac pacemakers, with electrodes stimulating the vagus nerve rather than the heart..

Sudarshan Kriya Yoga (SKY) emphasizes four breathing techniques that stimulate the vagus nerve. SKY has been studied in severely depressed people and has been found to be extremely effective at treating depressed mood. SKY and a simplified version called Breath Water Sound (BWS) were taught to survivors of the 2004 tsunami in Southeast Asia and the victims of Hurricane Katrina in 2005, and these interventions were found to be powerfully effective in reducing symptoms of posttraumatic stress disorder.

The way that yoga is practiced, focusing your mind on your own body, concentrating on your physical being (some positions are very difficult and require intense effort), and carefully manipulating your breathing patterns, you become entirely focused on the here-and-now. This is completely opposite to the way people normally operate when they are anxious, either ruminating about problems from the past or worrying about the future. Rarely do people let go of these thoughts and simply look at themselves just at the present moment in time. Previously, I discussed the concept of letting go and strategies of relaxation aimed at relieving you of past and future worries. Yoga is one of many ways to achieve this state of mind.

Whether you believe in the spiritual aspects of yoga, are intrigued by its physiological effects on the brain, or are just generally curious about the practice, I encourage you to try it. Many people practice yoga, and even without understanding the "real" way that it causes change in them, they leave feeling strangely peaceful and relaxed. Some report feeling euphoric. In a study of patients with severe depression who required hospitalization, those who were randomly assigned to receive an intensive twenty-two-hour training in SKY were found to improve as well as the others, who were randomly assigned to receive conventional antidepressant medication.

Since the biological effects of yoga are real, it should not be taken lightly. Women who are pregnant and people who have medical conditions, such as uncontrolled high blood pressure, seizure disorder, significant heart disease, recent injuries or surgery, or any other serious medical illness, should consult his or her physician before considering a yoga program. Bipolar disorder and psychotic disorders such as schizophrenia may be worsened by SKY breathing techniques.

If you decide to try yoga, be aware that at this time there are no standard certification or licensure requirements to be a yoga instructor, though many instructors attend yoga institutes, where they are certified after completing a training program. Certification by the larger yoga centers usually requires at least 200 hours of teaching experience, daily practice of yoga for six months, total abstinence from alcohol and other drugs, and adherence to a strict vegetarian diet; obtaining certification from these training programs therefore demonstrates a high degree of personal dedication and experience in yoga. Nonetheless, keep in mind that there is no regulation of the quality of education at yoga schools. Until clearer standards are set, make sure that your yoga instructor is at least certified by a yoga school, and observe a class before deciding if you are comfortable participating in it.

Massage

Massage sounds like an indulgence rather than a health-maintenance activity. The Protestant work ethic that is considered the basis of American culture trains us to believe that truly good things can be achieved only through hard work, not pleasure. We still feel the influence of this old work ethic today, a good example being the expression "no pain, no gain," which became popular in the 1980s. However, there are some enjoyable and indulgent activities that can also be good for you, such as massage.

There are various schools of massage. Examples include Swedish massage, deep tissue massage, sports/medical massage, *qi gong*, shiatsu, and

Thai massage, among many others. Each has its own theory as to why it is effective. However, they all have something in common: in some way they physically "force" your muscles into a state of relaxation. While meditation tries to achieve a relaxed state from within (the mind), massage complements this by physically "forcing" a relaxed state from without (the body).

It can be astounding how much stress, tension, or emotion we hold in our muscles. People with stress commonly suffer from stiff necks, backaches, or tension headaches. I first became truly aware of how much tension and emotion our muscles hold after the terrorist attacks on September 11, 2001. The American Red Cross set up a vast disaster relief service center in New York for all people affected by the disaster. Volunteer services ranged widely, including medical and psychiatric evaluations, legal assistance, and provision of various social services. Among the many disciplines was a large group of volunteer massage therapists. Many people tried massage, seeking comfort and stress relief. Others timidly requested massages, thinking that they would take advantage of a good opportunity for a free massage, while they had come to the Red Cross Center to find help for someone else. The response of all people, regardless of why they came, was dramatic. Some of those who had come for others' sake and who had thought they were strong and unaffected by the attacks found themselves in tears in the middle of a massage session. They had been holding in so much stress that the massage literally kneaded out the pent-up feelings. When I witnessed this, I realized how powerful a tool massage could really be.

Unlike yoga, massage therapy is regulated by each state government, requiring specific training and licensure. However, there are so many styles of massage, and the experience of touch is so unique, that you can have a completely different experience from two licensed massage therapists practicing for the same length of time. Make sure your massage therapist is licensed. Ask what kinds of massage techniques he or she uses and how long he or she has been practicing. If the response to these questions is vague, find another therapist—anyone who is truly trained and licensed would be able to answer these questions in detail. Consider what kind of massage would be more relaxing—the more superficial Swedish massage (which can still be vigorous depending on the massage therapist) or the much harder and sometimes painful deep-tissue massage. Pick a therapist with a gender you are most comfortable with—this is a nonsexual experience, and your comfort with the therapist is essential for the massage to reduce your stress. And don't make assumptions about gender and the strength of the massage—some women give powerfully deep massages, and some men have a more superficial style. Specify what you are looking for when you speak with a potential massage therapist. And most important, if you have had any kind of injury, recent surgery, or illness check with your physician to see if massage is safe for you

Acupuncture

Acupuncture is an East Asian medical treatment based on a perspective of the body that is completely different from that of Western medicine. While there are many schools of acupuncture, they all share a fundamental belief that the body is made up of a series of meridians, or channels for energy called qi (pronounced "chee"). In addition, they believe that the body is governed by two opposing universal forces: yin and yang. They complement each other, and when one is deficient or in excess, the body is not balanced, resulting in poor function. According to the teachings of traditional Eastern medicine, illnesses, including pain, stress, and addiction, stem from blockages of qi and imbalances of yin and yang. Hair-thin needles are inserted at points along these meridians to open up blockages and improve energy flow. In modern acupuncture, sometimes small amounts of electricity are even used to stimulate the energy channels though the needles. Correcting the flow of energy in your body using acupuncture and balancing yin and yang through diet and other lifestyle changes, along with other eastern remedies, can help restore you to health. Many people report leaving an acupuncture session feeling relaxed and tranquil, with a general sense of well-being.

Western medicine has tried to make sense of acupuncture, explaining it with the principles of Western medicine, such as finding nerve pathways that may be directly stimulated by the needles. However, these studies have not been able to explain adequately all the things that acupuncture is capable of doing. In some extraordinary cases, acupuncture has been used as an anesthetic in surgery, without the use of any pain medications. However, acupuncture is considered to be most useful in improving milder ailments by achieving balance in the body and leaving the patient with a sense of overall well-being. Acupuncture has been found to be particularly helpful with certain pain syndromes, addiction, anxiety, high blood pressure, digestive problems, and even hemorrhoids. However, for major medical illnesses, I strongly advise patients to use Western medicine, consider acupuncture as an adjuvant treatment. Even in East Asia, where acupuncture was developed, most doctors and common people believe that it is best used in conjunction with Western medicine, with each complementing the other.

Some people respond very dramatically to acupuncture, while others may not have much response at all. Some studies completely debunk any therapeutic value to acupuncture, though this goes against the positive experiences of millions of people. Some studies that find validity in the treatment have also found that if acupuncture has not shown any benefit after three to four treatments, the statistical chance of any improvement with continued acupuncture is extremely small. In that case, it is time to try a different relaxation strategy.

Acupuncture is also a practice that is regulated by state governments, requiring licenses to practice. If you try acupuncture, make sure that the practitioner is licensed in your state and always uses brand-new needles that are individually, sterilely wrapped. In general, acupuncture by itself is extremely safe and surprisingly painless and soothing. If the acupuncturist recommends herbal remedies in addition to the acupuncture, be cautious and discuss this with your physician first, as they can be just as powerful as pharmaceutical medicines and drugs (remember that cocaine, marijuana, heroin, and opium are all from plants) and may chemically trigger a relapse or interact with medications that you are already taking.

Reiki

Reiki is both an ancient and a new form of holistic healing with roots dating back several thousands of years in Tibet. It is a system of healing that involves the placement of hands directly on the recipient, as well as holding one's hands near the recipient's body without any actual physical contact. The "laying on of hands" as a treatment for ailments has existed throughout history in various cultures, even in Christian fundamentalist groups in the United States, so it is difficult to know the true origin of Reiki. A Japanese educator named Dr. Mikao Usui developed the modern practice of Reiki in the late 1800s, looking for a spiritual system of healing through study, research, and meditation. He reported that at one point, he experienced a metaphysical transformation, and based on that experience he developed a system of healing using what he called the "Universal Life Force," which is channeled into a recipient's body. Ailments are conceptualized as an obstruction of the flow of the Universal Life Force, and the Reiki practitioner acts as a conduit to direct the energy back into the recipient.

By tradition, the Reiki healing system was passed down from master to disciple in Japan. However, all of the original masters in Japan died, except for one master, who immigrated to Hawaii, where she continued to teach Reiki to Americans. For this reason, Reiki is now more developed and widely practiced as a healing art in the United States than it is in Japan.

Anecdotally, many people have reported unusual experiences with Reiki, including stimulation of bowel activity, heavy salivation, muscle twitches, or unusual body sensations, even when there is no physical contact with the Reiki healer. Some people simply leave a session feeling a deeper sense of calm. Some people do not notice any effect at all.

While extreme Reiki enthusiasts believe that Reiki can heal almost any physical ailment, many people, including some Reiki practitioners, feel that its greatest use is for relaxation, which in turn improves overall health. I do not recommend that people use Reiki as a primary treatment for any medical condition. However, effective relaxation techniques are good complementary treatments for almost all medical conditions because stress has such a pervasive negative impact on the entire body. While massage may be wonderful for some people, it may be inappropriate for people with certain physical injuries or people who feel more anxious from too much physical contact. In this regard, Reiki may be a nice alternative, with minimal to no physical contact.

Meditation

Meditation is defined by Merriam Webster's Dictionary as focusing the mind or pondering in self-reflection. There are many practices that would fall under this definition, such as prayer, Transcendental Meditation, Buddhist chanting, Zen meditation, and even sitting in a comfortable chair at home focusing on colorful fish in an aquarium.

Because meditation can be done in so many ways, the best kind is whatever method fits your personality, lifestyle, and personal philosophy. Your goal is to feel more tranquil, so finding a good fit, like the right size shoes, will make the difference between a comfortable, relaxing experience, in which you can clear your mind, and an uncomfortable and self-conscious activity in which your mind is preoccupied with your discomfort. Do whatever feels good to you.

EXERCISE 17-1 MEDITATION ROUTINE

THIS meditation exercise combines aspects of many different meditation and relaxation techniques. Try to do this exercise twice a day—once in the morning to start the day in a tranquil state of mind, and once in the evening to help yourself unwind from the stresses of the day. Allow yourself 5 to 10 minutes each time you do this. If you cannot spare 5 to 10 minutes to devote to your own well-being twice a day, you've identified a significant problem right there!

Find a comfortable, dark, and quiet place to sit or lie down and close your eyes. The first time you do this, you may want someone else with a calming voice to read you these instructions and guide you through the steps.

1. Sit or lie comfortably with your eyes closed. If you are lying down, lay your arms and hands at your sides. If you are sitting, place the palms of your hands on the tops of your thighs.
2. Take note of your body, its position in the chair or on the bed, how it feels lying against the cushions. If you are sitting, feel the sensation of the palms of your hands resting on your thighs.
3. Shift your attention to your neck and your shoulders and note how they feel. Imagine they are made of lead, and let them drop. Notice how you may have been tensing them and holding them up, and try to appreciate their heaviness as you let them fully relax.
4. Take in a slow deep breath through your mouth over 5 seconds, then exhale slowly through your nose over 5 seconds.

5. Take in another slow deep breath and visualize the air coming in through your mouth and filling your lungs. Imagine it as white steam or vapor, filling every pocket and opening in your lungs, and be aware of your lungs gradually expanding and filling with air.

6. Slowly exhale through your nose and visualize the air coming out in streams of slightly grayish vapor from your nostrils, carrying out any bad feelings, stress, tension, and "impurities"—the grayish tinge—that you have stored inside you.

7. Repeat this deep breathing and visualization a total of 5 times.

8. After completing 5 cycles of deep breathing, repeat the following words out loud, thinking deeply about their meanings as you say them:

Just for today,
   I do not need to get angry.
   I do not need to worry.
   I will be grateful for what I have.
   I will work hard.
   I will be kind to others.

9. After saying these statements, repeat the deep breathing again for 5 more breaths

10. Slowly count backward from 10 to 1, and when you reach 1, slowly open your eyes. Now you are done.

WHO IS IN YOUR SOCIAL CIRCLE?

Dealing with Loneliness
and Finding a Sober Group of Friends

IF YOU ARE trying to stop crystal but most of your friends still use it, as well as other drugs, you have an extra challenge in trying to stay sober. Remember the mantra "people, places, and things" reminding you that the people you associate with crystal are dangerous because they can easily pull you back into using again. People who used crystal in private—hidden from family and friends, doing meth only with strangers, sex hookups, and their dealer—may still know several sober people who are not triggers and who can support them through their efforts to stay clean.

But what if your main social circle is a group of other drug users, people with whom you used to spend most of your free time, whether it was just hanging out at home getting high or going out together to parties where everyone was using drugs. What if you are a gay man, and your social circle is all circuit boys who talk mostly about clubs, the best DJs, and what drugs they plan to do for the weekend? If any of these resembles your situation, then trying to separate yourself from these people can be difficult because it means giving up your entire social network, the people you are accustomed to calling whenever you are bored, lonely, or looking for something to do. If you have to cut ties with these people, then how are you going to make it through each day?

Whoever you are, and however you identify yourself, it is essential to understand the *personal* significance of your own social group. Who are the people in your social circle of drug users and why are they so important? Whether gay or straight, ask yourself this question and consider whether other people can meet these same needs. If you are a straight young man in a small rural town and just out of high school, you may have a core group of friends you know from school. You've been friends since freshman year, which feels like a lifetime, and in your small town there don't seem to be many people to choose for friends. But are there really no other people, or is it just easier to keep hanging with the same crew you always did? Unless you and your friends were the only people in your graduating class, there are probably other people that are potential friends. The easiest way to meet sober friends is to go to the nearest twelve-step meeting. Even if you aren't exactly the same age, you may find that you have more important things in common than your age, especially your wish to stay clean!

If you are a gay man in the club/circuit scene, believe it or not, there are other fun, attractive, and gay-affirming people in the world who do not use drugs, and they can offer you the same support you had from your party friends. In fact, they can probably offer you even better support because they may be more interested in the person you are, unlike many club friends whose main concern is whether you are have any E and K to share or if you're going to give Tina a call this weekend.

Gay men who were introduced to the party scene when they were just coming out may have an even greater challenge separating from their social group. Before coming out, they may have been completely closeted and unable to be their true selves with anyone. Alternatively, their peers may have known they were gay and ostracized them, making them feel they were worthless outcasts. The group of partying friends may be the first people ever to fully accept them, the first to make them feel liked and to welcome them into their group. More than just people with whom they are accustomed to passing time and doing drugs, these friends have strong, positive emotional meaning in these men's lives.

Similarly, circuit parties, which are huge gatherings with thousands of gay men, most of them high on club drugs, are places where many gay men first felt they could openly and wholeheartedly celebrate their sexuality, feeling happy, attractive, and accepted into a community. The feeling of being surrounded by a sea of gay men contrasts so sharply to the feeling of isolation from their closeted pasts. Therefore, the entire scene—the friends, the parties, and the drugs—has a monumental emotional significance to these men.

Asking these gay men to stop seeing their party friends and to stop going to circuit parties is asking them to turn their backs on the first people who made them feel accepted and not to go back to the place where they remember first truly feeling part of a community. While all these fond memories have some validity, in reality, drugs were likely the real glue that held much of this group together, and ultimately, the drugs and sex became the main draws to the circuit parties. The positive associations to these people and places are so deep that it can be incredibly difficult to let go. As positive as their feelings may be, however, this group of friends who once seemed like a lifeline gradually turned into a ball and chain dragging them to a drowning death by crystal addiction.

If these gay ex–party boys have no significant friends outside the club and circuit scene, then completely separating themselves from this social scene will bring on a period of profound loneliness and isolation. They will need a strong support system (including their drug counselor, therapist, twelve-step groups, other recovery groups, and any sober family and friends who are willing to help) to maintain their motivation to stay clean while they explore ways of meeting new, sober gay friends who share a bond with them other than drugs. If they make it through this period, they will discover what it is like to have gay friends who truly like them for who they are, not just because they do drugs together at parties.

If you are an offbeat club kid, marginalized at school as "that strange chick," but considered "the cool, cute babe" in the rave scene, you may be surprised to find other teens like you who swim outside the mainstream but still think they are cool, and are clean and sober. When you hear the obnoxious Barbies at school make fun of your different clothes, if you stop going to raves, where the scene and the drugs remind you that you are still that cute, cool, babe—now you are forced to look at how you really feel about yourself and admit how much of an effect those vicious girls at school really had on your self-image. You felt cool at the rave parties, but if you can't go back to the scene, will the cool babe you were at the parties magically disappear, or will she still be inside you somewhere?

Hold on to the pride and self-esteem you remember from the parties, but don't resort to club drugs to erase the nasty words of the Barbies. It will be a hard struggle, but learning that you're still cool, no matter what those girls say, shows how powerless the Barbies really are. Now you've developed *real* personal strength and confidence—and you don't need meth to chemically brainwash you into believing it. A lot of the teens at raves are in the exact same situation you are. Some of them are stuck on rolling and are too addicted to stop the partying. But you may find some who are willing to forage outside the rave scene to see if they can still feel good about themselves without the drugs. If none of your rave friends can see things the way you do, go to a teen AA meeting, and you'll find many young people just like you. The friends you make there will share your desire to stay clean and will also join you in the process of finding the cool, cute babe inside each of you.

TAKING THE FIRST STEP

BEFORE TACKLING THE seemingly impossible notion of leaving your friends forever, first tell yourself that you need some space from everyone and everything associated with crystal, at least for *right now*. This is a much easier time frame to grasp. It may mean this week, it may mean the next several weeks. You cannot give yourself a definite date, but you know that right now you are not able be around people or places that will tempt you to use crystal. During that time, work on stopping crystal completely and getting stronger supports that will help you stay clean—non–drug-using friends, close family members, a drug counselor, a therapist, or a drug treatment program.

Once you have detoxed from crystal and made these connections, work on developing relapse prevention skills, so that if you see your old friends, you will be better prepared to deal with tempting situations and the strong feelings they will bring up. For example, practice refusal skills especially when you know that old friends are going to try to get you to use. Design your own mental exercises tailored to what situations you imagine you will be in, and practice them again and again to help you resist the urge to use if you know that your friends will still be using around you.

WHAT IF YOU KEEP USING WITH YOUR FRIENDS?

IF SEEING YOUR friends who use crystal or other drugs eventually pulls you back into using, then you have the difficult task of assessing how these people fit into your life. If you keep relapsing in their company, then they are literally pulling you down a life-threatening spiral of addiction.

This does not necessarily mean your friends are "bad" people. It simply means that being with them results in an unhealthy situation that is dangerous for you. Again, consider the asthma analogy—suppose you had asthma and an allergy to cats, and you walk into a room with a litter of five adorable kittens. They are cute and fuzzy, asking you for affection and love. Despite how cute and affectionate they are, being with them will trigger an allergic reaction and a severe asthma attack that could land you in the hospital—you know this from previous experiences with cats. The kittens are not bad per se, but being near them is dangerous, and you need to stay away from them. This is how you should view your drug-using friends—without judgment but with clear acknowledgment of the risk they pose to you.

Once you are sober and are committed to stopping crystal, you may find that with drugs out of the picture, you have a lot less in common with your old friends than you had thought. Drugs and the activities associated with them often form the fundamental bond that brings many people together. While it may seem that there are other reasons that you are friends, drug use may be the most significant reason. It's only when you stop using meth that its role in your friendship becomes clearer. Which do your friends seem more concerned about—protecting your health or the next time they are going to do meth?

Finding "Sober Friends" JUSTIN'S STORY

Justin became such a recluse, staying in his room doing crystal, that he couldn't work, and he ran out of money to pay for the drug, even though his friend made it and sold it to him very cheaply. He also started to become paranoid and suspicious about his friend. To avoid dealing with him, he decided to try making his own crystal, using the recipe his friend had found on the Internet.

The state Justin lived in was cracking down hard on small, hidden meth labs. One day two police cars drove up and uncovered Justin's secret lab. They arrested him, and he was convicted of manufacturing illegal substances.

Justin was sentenced to prison, where he was treated by the prison psychiatrist for his psychotic paranoia and hallucinations. Justin's prison time was shortened with the stipulation that he participate in a court-mandated residential drug-treatment program in a town one hour from his home. After completing the program, he was clean from meth for two years.

Justin returned home to an empty house—his mother had moved in with a new boyfriend. He resumed his life where he had left off, working at a gas station part time. He was happy to see his old friends again, no longer paranoid and suspicious of them. However, they were still using meth, smoking it to while away their free time. When he first saw them high after he had been clean for so long, Justin didn't like what he saw and realized how far he had let himself go. He had an even stronger resolve not to start crystal again.

After two months back at home, Justin was still clean. He wanted to stay away from crystal, but it was difficult. He didn't know anyone else to hang out with, because his community was so small—it was difficult to meet new people that he liked. With only a part-time job to keep him busy, he soon found himself in the same dilemma as before—having nothing to do, he felt bored and "useless." He started having strong memories of the excitement he felt when using crystal—not just mental images but even bodily sensations. All he could focus on was how everything felt so vibrant and interesting when he was high. Though he also recalled the anxiety, paranoia, and malnutrition that he had suffered, it seemed like a faded memory in comparison to the strong, visceral feelings of how good it felt to be high. Eventually the draw became overwhelming, and one day when he was hanging out with his friends while they were smoking crystal, he asked them to pass him the pipe. They were surprised but happy to have their old friend back in the fold and relieved not to have a teetotaler hovering around them, making them feel judged and uncomfortable about their drug use.

Justin started with just doing crystal on his days off from work, but within a month he was smoking every day again, and soon his paranoia and hallucinations returned. Fortunately, he recognized what was happening to him, especially when he started hearing voices again. He still had the telephone number of the drug treatment facility he had gone to after prison, and he called his old counselor. Justin returned to rehab.

During his second rehab, Justin had even more material to talk about with his counselor and with the groups, looking at what exactly caused him to relapse. He discussed his boredom and the lack of structure to most of his days, which intensified his cravings. He complained about how difficult it was to find friends who didn't use meth, making excuses for why he kept hanging out with people who were smoking right in front of him. Even though he had talked about these same issues during his first rehab, he didn't really connect with the discussions until he experienced them firsthand when he returned home.

During Justin's second rehab, he had more motivation and insight, and he worked closely with his counselor to develop a plan for what he would do after discharge: he realized that even though his community was small, there were places in his town where he could find potential friends. He had dismissed those people because he assumed that because they were not drug users, they must be boring. But now they seemed like safer options, which was comforting as he began to understand that his old "interesting" friends were actually dangerous to him. As paranoid and psychotic as he had gotten, his friends kept smoking meth in front of him while he struggled not to use so that he would never have to hear those terrifying voices in his head again. He left rehab with a new desire to make sober friends with whom he could stay clean.

Justin found an AA meeting that was in a town one hour away. There were no CMA meetings in his area, but a group recovering from alcoholism was close enough—he could still talk about addiction and get support from other people trying to get sober. He was surprised to find another person from his community at one of the meetings, and they become "sober friends." Now, when Justin felt lonely he did not have to call his old drug-using friends anymore.

Even though the AA meetings were an hour away by car, he went to the meetings every day that he was not working at the gas station, and even on some days after he finished work. He had a more regular schedule, and life didn't seem so formless and lacking in direction. While he regretted not having a better job, he felt he was working hard to move forward, and he felt more empowered. He had something to feel proud about.

Justin still struggles with bouts of strong urges to use crystal, especially when he feels disappointed with himself and frustrated with his life. However, whenever he feels this way, he calls his sponsor or one of his sober friends. When cravings are intense, he goes to town and waits for the next AA meeting. None of his old friends cook meth anymore because all the local basement labs were shut down by the police. Still, Justin heard that crystal was available in town from an outside source, but he has resisted asking about it so that there is no possibility he can find any crystal if his temptation to use becomes irresistible. Eighteen months have passed since Justin last used crystal, and he is still struggles with occasional cravings, but he "fights the good fight" and remains motivated.

A SOCIAL EXPERIMENT

SEE WHAT HAPPENS when you spend time with your friends and do not use drugs. In this experiment, I refer to any drug except alcohol. That includes Ecstasy, marijuana, cocaine, Special K, and crystal, as well as any other illicit substance or even prescription medications, such as OxyContin, that are not used according to the medical instructions. Consider yourself the investigator of this small sociology experiment. The purpose of the study is to observe what happens to a group of friends who regularly use club drugs together, when one person decides that, for health reasons, he or she wants to stay away from all drugs. During the experiment, the designated sober person steadfastly refuses all drugs for two weeks (at least two cycles of weekend partying), while the others are free to choose whatever they want to do.

You are the sober person in this experiment—remember that you must remain completely sober for the experiment to work. Focus your attention on what happens among the group members while you remain sober. Note but try not to dwell on the nagging feeling that if you just did a little crystal, or even just a tab of E or a bump of K while the rest of your friends were partying, your interactions would be much more comfortable. In fact, the discomfort you notice is one of the things you are trying to understand in this study. This exercise requires you to step outside yourself and look at the entire group, including yourself, as if you were an outside observer. This will give you a more accurate picture of what happens to the group, and by intellectually removing yourself from the situation, it may be easier to emotionally step back, rather than to get caught up in the powerful emotions that could push you back into using drugs. If you are able to complete this exercise, you will learn important things about yourself and your friends, and you may make some significant changes in your friendships and your life.

If you are fortunate during the time that you remain completely sober, you may discover that there are many non–drug-related activities that you enjoy doing with your friends. Maybe you already knew this, but perhaps your friends realized they could enjoy themselves together without necessarily using drugs. Your friends must also be sober when engaging in these activities with you. Participating in activities and connecting with each other *without* any drugs, you may form deeper, more meaningful friendships that are not distorted by chemical highs—anyone can be fun to hang out with if you take the right drug, but if you need drugs to tolerate someone, perhaps that's not a good person for you to be around.

On the other hand, you may find it difficult or awkward to relate to these friends without using drugs. Some people in your social circle may be uncomfortable, feeling that you are judging their drug use: "If he thinks it's bad for him, he must think I'm bad for doing it." You may also find some friends who keep pushing you to do drugs, even after you've told them repeatedly that you don't want to. After so many refusals, why do they keep pushing? Do they have any respect for your wish to stay clean? How important to them is your health, which you are trying to protect from drug use? Or do they even care about your desires, clearly repeated several times? How do their concerns about you compare to their need to get you to do drugs with them? Some people need to have others use drugs with them because it makes the act seem more acceptable —they are helping *themselves* feel less guilty about their own drug use. Does this need to justify their own drug use overshadow their concern for you and their respect for your wishes?

You may find that when you take drugs out of your friendships, there is little else left that you actually have in common. *When Boys Fly* is a documentary that follows four very different gay men as they go to the same circuit party. One young man promises his roommate at home that at the circuit party he will not use drugs because, despite serious problems with drugs in the past, he is determined to prove that he does not have a problem with drugs, and that circuit parties are not just about drugs. They are spiritual and communal experiences for gay men. Before arriving at the party, he tells the camera about his "closest friend," a slightly older man who he says understands him deeply, better than anyone else in the world. The friend is a "circuit buddy," someone he only sees when he goes to circuit parties around the country. The two run into each other only briefly every couple of months at circuit parties when they are both high. Nonetheless, the earnest young man firmly believes the two are soul mates. After a long, frustrating search among thousands of men, he finally finds his friend. The young man is sober and jumping with excitement but the friend is almost mute, staring with a smiling yet empty expression, with glazed eyes as large as saucers. It is clear to the viewer that something does not match. While the young man is jumping with glee, his "closest friend in the world" appears frozen, almost without any reaction. The viewer wonders what actually makes these two men so close. Only after the young man breaks his promise and starts using drugs do the two "friends" relate in any significant way—the old friendship is rekindled. So is it really friendship, or are drugs the real bond that connects these two?

When you consider the friendship in this documentary, you may realize that some of the people in your own life may just be drug friends. When you first join a group of partyers, big differences may seem like a positive thing—"Wow, I've developed a group of really diverse friends from all different backgrounds!" However, when you try to sustain some of these relationships *without* drugs, it becomes clear which relationships are based on drugs and which have real substance. Consider carefully how you define a "friend." Then think about which people in your group of partyers fit this definition. If these people are not really your friends, and they are putting you at risk for relapsing, you need to let go and move on.

Socializing in circles of drug-using friends makes it easy to always have people around you. Drug users consciously or unconsciously find each other, quietly assessing people and asking themselves, "Is he one of us or not? Does he even know what Tina is?" The ease of finding drug friends is extremely attractive because it wards off loneliness. The temptation to fall back on this group can be strong if you are alone and trying to find a new group of friends who are sober. Forming friendships based on something real can take much longer than friendships based on drugs. But patience and hard work pay off because you will develop real friendships with people who have a real connection to you, rather than an artificial semblance of a friend that is really just another excuse to use drugs, disguised in human form.

LETTING GO

LETTING GO of drug-using friends is a difficult but necessary task for successful recovery. If these people are your primary friends, you are making a tremendous sacrifice, much more than just crystal—you are giving up your main social network and your usual social support system.

Gay men living closeted lives in homophobic areas of the country may look to their drug-using club/circuit friends as their supportive brothers and their only connection to the gay community. It may be difficult to believe that they can find many other gay men who are sober, whether they simply do not use drugs or are ex-partyers like themselves who are in recovery. In fact, sober friends would likely be even better supports, possibly being more available to you when you really need help, not just when you are looking to have fun and party.

Drug users in general, male or female, gay or straight, are part of a drug culture, and the underground nature of illicit drug use gives drug users a common bond. For those drug users who don't feel connected to any other group, the sense of belonging to the drug community can be difficult to let go.

For people who live in small communities in rural areas, where meeting strangers is rare, the prospect of giving up the few close friends they have now is even more daunting because it seems as if there may be no one—sober or not—to replace them.

Regardless of which group you fall into, the idea of cutting off contact with your main social group can be frightening. For this reason, it is extremely helpful to get connected with treatment, whether with a therapist, a drug counselor, a twelve-step group, or other support groups.

Your sober network will provide you with supportive backup while you test out your old friendships with your new sober life, help you to assess whether you need to end certain harmful friendships, give you the skills and courage to break away from old destructive relationships, and be there for you to give you support when you finally let go.

Letting go of your old friends can feel incredibly lonely. In contrast to having a large group of meth-using friends who were always available to party, you may feel extremely alone during your search for new friends. However, building a new circle is very possible, though it requires some effort. If you are recently coming off crystal, you may feel down, socially withdrawn, and not at all interested in reaching out to new people right now. Others may crave connection and want some handholding through this difficult stage of early sobriety. No matter what your situation, you should reach out for support because remaining isolated puts you at risk for relapsing. If you feel withdrawn right now, at the very least, use your sober treatment supports (AA, CMA, drug counselors, therapists, and so on) to maintain healthy contact with the outside world while you gradually develop a new circle of friends.

YOUR NEW FRIENDS

THE NOTION OF finding a whole new group of people to get to know, trust, and open yourself up to, as well as finding people that you would actually enjoy spending time with, sounds monumental if you are starting from scratch. However, this is something that most people go through, and they do it successfully. This is a normal part of life, even outside the addiction world. Take for example people who move to another town in a distant state for a new job. The initial transition is difficult, but eventually they find new friends.

Let me reemphasize the importance of utilizing your relapse prevention network to maintain some healthy social contact during this period so you do not feel completely cut off. Loneliness and boredom can be strong triggers that draw you back to meth. In addition, the frustration of feeling socially disconnected when you are used to the ease of old friends constantly within reach will create a great temptation to go back to your old group.

For the time being, CMA, other twelve-step organizations such as AA or NA, or a non–twelve-step support group can be your temporary social circle. A therapist can serve as a confidant with whom you can share your difficulties as well as your triumphs and joys. A twelve-step sponsor can be there for you to call at any time if you need someone to speak to immediately. You may find that some of the people in this "surrogate" social circle become good friends, sharing many things in common with you, especially the difficult task of sobriety and all the obstacles that come along the way.

The process of making new friends may be gradual and take a long time. As frustrating as it may feel, this is actually a great opportunity to significantly improve your life. Take the time to think about what you *really* want from friendships, and make a list of what characteristics are most important to you. Your experience with "drug friends," an extreme version of fake friendships that happen to most people, taught you a lot about what makes a friendship satisfying and real. If you are prepared with your list of what you expect of real friends, whenever you meet someone, you have a better ability to assess how this person may fit into your life, and you can decide who you want to incorporate into your social network. Gradually, you will fill your life with healthier and more meaningful relationships.

Here are a few questions to think about when considering whether someone has the potential to be the kind of friend you want in your life:

- Is the person interesting?
- Do you have any things in common—experiences, hobbies, sense of humor?
- Is this person different, but in areas that you would like to learn more about?
- Is this person different, but is interested in learning more about you?
- Is this person so different that you both find it difficult to understand each other?
- Is this person caring and sympathetic?
- Can this person listen or is this person mostly a talker? Does he or she have the capacity to really listen when you need someone to talk to?
- Does the person ask about you, as well as talk about him- or herself?

- Does this person have the capacity to care about you, sympathize with you, or support you emotionally if you need help? Or does the person keep changing the direction of the conversation back to him- or herself?
- Does the person use drugs or is the person in recovery?
- Does this person seem like he or she can handle knowing that you are in recovery?
- Is this person trustworthy and dependable?

These are only a few examples of questions that you might ask. Think of other questions about the qualities that are most important and meaningful to you.

Making new friendships may not be as quick as it was when you were using crystal or other party drugs, when the common bond of the drugs was what brought people together easily. Dr. Edward Khantzian, a well-known psychoanalyst and addiction specialist, believed that the actual friendship was between the addict and the drug. *Crystal* was your real friend, and the people associated with it were objects that you and "Chrissie" used to enjoy your time together. In this light it is even clearer why it is so difficult to make new friends—it is as if you were married to someone for several years, during which you were no longer dating—the relationship turned bitterly destructive, so you divorced, and now you're back on the dating scene. But it's hard to put yourself out there and meet new people again. You feel lonely, awkward, and out of practice in the social scene. Also, when you meet new prospects, sometimes you remember the best things about your ex, and new relationships seem dull and dissatisfying in comparison. Divorced people often have rough starts, but eventually they start meeting new people again.

Sober people who would make good friends may be right under your nose. Non–crystal-using friends who had been in your life but who fell by the wayside during your crystal years may still be around, and they may be glad to hear of the return of the old friend they thought they had lost to drugs. Important relationships with family members may have grown distant, but hopefully not too far to reach and try to reconnect.

The Eighth Step in twelve-step programs is to make a list of all persons one has harmed, and become willing to make amends to them all. The Ninth Step is: "Make direct amends to such people wherever possible, except when to do so would injure them or others." "Persons we have harmed" include those that you may have rejected and broken ties with because of your addiction. The Eighth and Ninth Steps remind you of important people you may have lost as a result of crystal. They confront you with the ugly truth that your addiction damaged and potentially destroyed those relationships, and they give you an opportunity to repair them.

Developing new friendships now may feel different and much more difficult than earlier experiences because instead of adding new friends to your existing group, you may have to start completely from scratch. Keep a list of ideal qualities in mind when forming new friendships, but also remember that these qualities are not always apparent the first time your meet someone. You may have to meet a lot of people before you find any that seem even remotely "friend-worthy" according to your criteria. However, even with the "right" people, it takes time to get to know each other and to develop a trusting and caring bond—no one can meet all the requirements of your list at first meeting. Keep yourself open to different people, even those you might not have considered in the past, and try to stay optimistic. While you are getting to know people, always keep your wish list of criteria in mind. You may even decide to make changes as you meet more people and further clarify your definition of a satisfying friendship. If you get the sense that the person uses drugs, say good-bye immediately. You are in recovery and your health is too important. No matter how interesting that person seems, he or she poses a great risk to you. The crystal-craving part of your mind may sense the possibility that the person is a drug user, and unconsciously the person may seem even more appealing, because you know that spending time with that person will lead to using crystal again. Before this happens, if you start to feel this smallest possibility that the person uses drugs, stay away.

When first stopping crystal, you may not feel very sociable, especially during the acute withdrawal, which usually occurs one to seven days after stopping. However, depression and social withdrawal can linger for several weeks thereafter. If you feel this way, give yourself a break and for now, use your recovery network for social support and connection. After a month, if you are still feeling lonely but aren't getting yourself out of the house, force yourself out there. If you are really feeling stuck, see a psychiatrist to see if you are clinically depressed. Some symptoms of a biological depression, aside from low mood, include social withdrawal, feelings of hopelessness, low energy, and poor motivation—all of which can be keeping you stuck in a rut, preventing you from making new friends, and putting you at risk for relapsing on crystal. Appropriate treatment for depression can get you back on your feet and starting to rebuild your social network.

WHERE DO I FIND NEW PEOPLE?

KEEP YOURSELF OPEN to meeting people but try not to search so aggressively that your search becomes a hunting expedition. If you are relaxed and open to meeting new people, you can encounter potential friends in any place and at any time—on the street, when you are shopping, at work—any place you find yourself. Places to *avoid* meeting friends are wherever you know or suspect there is drug activity—bars, clubs, circuit parties, sex parties, raves, and so on.

In addition to relying on random events, you can be proactive in meeting people. Go to social events and parties with sober friends. Attend sober events held by twelve-step groups. Find out about organizations and activity groups in your local area that interest you, whether it is a pottery class, a hiking group, a book club, or a continuing education class, particularly classes that are interactive, such as conversational language groups (many are designed as social events) or studio art courses. Try several different avenues until you find one that really feels enjoyable. At the very least, even if you don't find a new friend, you will be doing an activity that interests you. The fact that the other people at those activities chose to be there means that they share at least one interest with you. Hopefully there will be people there that you may also like as friends.

Another avenue worth exploring is volunteer work. Find a cause that you believe in, whether it is helping the homeless, fighting the HIV epidemic, supporting your favorite political cause, helping to organize the local Walk for Breast Cancer, or whatever is meaningful to you. Picking a cause that holds strong personal significance to you may help you meet others who share not only an interest but a *passion*—perhaps the shared passion will reveal even more similarities that will make the person seem more interesting as a friend. Making a positive interpersonal connection and doing something personally meaningful are both activities that most consistently stimulate the parts of the brain involved with happiness—both psychologically and physiologically, you are improving your mood and your experience of living sober.

Just a side note about volunteer work: volunteering is wonderful because at the same time that you help others, you also improve yourself. Being productive in a way that clearly benefits others is associated with improved self-esteem. Additionally, by helping others, you cognitively redirect your attention away from yourself and your own troubles, and you remind yourself that other people are suffering as well. Many people in recovery choose to volunteer or even devote their careers to addiction services and helping other addicts to stay sober. They find that this kind of work helps to keep their own sobriety under better control by letting them witness the dangers of addiction without having to relive it themselves. It also requires them to constantly think of innovative strategies to help other people stay sober, and shows them the positive results of sobriety in the people that they help. Addiction work keeps one's relapse prevention skills honed and provides strong motivation and reinforcement to stay clean and sober.

19

CRYSTAL AND SEX:
If Sex on Crystal Is So Amazing, Is It Possible to Enjoy Sex Without It?

SEX ON CRYSTAL

FOR MANY CRYSTAL users, sex is their primary activity when they get high. One reason for such a close association between this particular drug and sex is that they both stimulate the dopamine-mediated mesolimbic pathway. As discussed earlier, stimulating this pathway is nature's way of tricking animals to repeat behaviors, such as sex and eating, that help the animal, and ultimately the entire species, survive. Therefore, when the mesolimbic pathway is so powerfully overstimulated by methamphetamine, the drive to have sex is also stimulated to a pathological extreme.

Libido and sexual pleasure on crystal is exponentially more intense than sober sex because the mesolimbic pathway is stimulated to an unnaturally high degree that it was never meant to reach. When they are high, people spend hours or even days searching for sex, having sex, or masturbating. The drive can feel like an insatiable hunger. Crystal makes erections difficult or impossible to achieve for most men, so in the past, users were usually the recipient of anal sex (aka the "bottom"). Since the advent of

Viagra and similar medications that facilitate erections, men on crystal can now perform both the penetrative and the receptive role in anal sex. Since both partners are now able to use crystal and have equally long-lasting sex drives, the duration of sexual activities has increased significantly, and sex hookups or sex parties can last from hours to days.

Within the gay community, sex clubs have seen a dramatic change in sexual behavior. Many patrons now stay at the clubs much longer than in the past because they remain high on crystal for long periods, and during extended binges some patrons stay over twenty-four hours. Some sex clubs have resorted to strictly enforcing time limits when patrons must leave or pay another entrance fee. In the past, it was hard to imagine people staying for more than eight hours in a sex club, but as long as there is a supply of crystal to fuel the sex, time can be almost limitless.

Safer-sex practices have also changed. Despite the dedicated efforts of outreach workers to educate people about HIV-transmission and provide free condoms, increasing numbers of people are having sex without condoms. Many patrons in gay sex clubs report that some men refuse to have sex with them with a condom. Even though the threat of HIV, hepatitis, and other sexually transmitted diseases are well known, concern about the health risks seems negligible compared to the compelling urgency to have more sex. When experiencing intense sex is the most important objective, "condoms just get in the way."

Here is an example of a personal ad on an Internet sex site for gay men that illustrates how crystal can affect the sex drive:

> Looking for guys between 18 and 50 hight and weight proportionate that PNP/SLAM occasionaly. preferably guys that "SLAM" Cause after I "SLAM" all Ill wanna do is suck cock and get fucked over and over draining load after load of cum into my ass and mouth!!!
>
> [PNP = "party and play"—using crystal and having sex; SLAM = injecting drugs intravenously]

The following anecdotal report from a suburban emergency room is another illustration of how disturbingly pathological sexual compulsions can be when fueled by crystal:

Kevin **is a twenty-seven-year-old** heterosexual male who was taken to his local emergency room by his roommate. He was extremely agitated and presented with bleeding abrasions (worn-down skin) on his penis. Because he was so agitated and his pupils appeared dilated, a urine drug screen was performed and tested positive for methamphetamine. He admitted to the ER physician that he had been smoking meth and then masturbated for six hours, resulting in serious abrasions and tears in the skin on all surfaces of the shaft of his penis. Prior to that evening, the patient had only used methamphetamine intranasally, but that night was his first experience smoking it.

Prior to the night of this ER visit, Kevin used to snort crystal alone in his room because it often made him sexually preoccupied. His usual routine was to masturbate while watching pornographic videos for a couple of hours. Then if he still felt sexual, he would go to a bar to try to pick up a woman for sex. He was curious about smoking because his friends recently changed from snorting to smoking, and they said it was so much better. Because Kevin became so sexually preoccupied just from snorting, he wondered how he would feel smoking meth, but was terrified of embarrassing himself in front of his friends. They didn't become fixated on sex with the same intensity as Kevin. Usually while smoking they sat around joking until they became restless enough to take their cars to a large empty parking lot, where they drove wildly in figure eights.

That night Kevin felt particularly curious and borrowed his friend's glass pipe. Alone in the privacy of his room he tried smoking meth for the first time, and he found his sexual desire was far stronger than he had ever imagined it could be. He had taken 200 mg of Viagra (four times the average dose) so that he could maintain an erection while masturbating. He was engrossed in watching his video, stopping every fifteen minutes take another hit from the pipe. After each orgasm, it was more difficult to achieve the next, so his masturbating became more and more aggressive. Kevin was using a lotion containing alcohol, and some time after his third orgasm, he felt a burning sensation on his penis. He realized that they were little patches on his penis that were irritated from the constant rubbing. He just changed to a different lotion without alcohol and resumed where he had left off. After his fifth orgasm, it was extremely difficult to achieve another, but he compulsively smoked more crystal, and masturbated with even more determination, trying to have one more orgasm. After a total of six hours of smoking and masturbating, Kevin ran out of meth, and over the next ten to fifteen minutes, the compulsive drive to masturbate gradually waned. He felt increasingly tired and irritable, and he was becoming more aware of pain all over his penis. He looked down, and saw that the lotion on his hand and on his penis was streaked with blood. He had been so preoccupied with watching the video and trying to have an orgasm that he didn't notice that the irritated spots were starting to bleed or that he'd rubbed off some superficial layers of skin, leaving some patches of skin pink and raw. An hour after he had smoked the last of his meth, the discomfort in his penis had turned into excruciating, burning pain. When he started screaming, his roommate ran in, dressed him, and rushed him immediately to the emergency room.

While these reports sound disturbing to the outsider, people who combine crystal and sex often report it to be one of the most amazing experiences in their lives, and they long to repeat it. For some people, crystal sex feels so amazing that, in comparison, sober sex seems dull and unfulfilling. Many gay men start using crystal as an occasional way to spice up sex, but they find themselves relying on it more often, and some of them reach a point where they are unable to have sex without it. If you are trying stay meth-free, but crystal had become a necessary part of sex for you, it will be an extremely powerful trigger. Because sexual desire is a natural occurrence, this trigger is unavoidable, so the issue of sex and how you will deal with it must be thoroughly addressed.

BIDDING FAREWELL TO SEX ON CRYSTAL

LIFE WITHOUT CRYSTAL means life without crystal sex. It's that simple.

Many people who used to combine sex and meth recall intense, aggressive, compulsive, limit-pushing, cathartic, nonstop-pleasure sex marathons that they long for again, But having crystal sex means putting meth in your body at least one more time, something you can't afford to do. Once that happens, you know it won't be just a one-time indulgence. It can quickly spin into a full relapse that brings you right back into the full grip of addiction.

If your mind keeps going back to crystal sex, don't try to ignore it and pretend it never happened. The memory only fights harder to come back until you acknowledge it, and it may grow in power as the memories become even more idealized, like a little child calling out to you, jumping up and down, screaming louder and louder because he can't get your attention. It's all right to acknowledge this—but as a very special memory. You can recall it as an amazing time, like a trip to Antarctica with breathtaking sunrises over colossal glistening snow peaks, unlike anything you could see elsewhere on this planet—it was a grueling trek to get there, extremely expensive to arrange. You drove, camped, and hiked through temperatures 20 degrees below zero with fifty-mile-per-hour gusts or wind that gave your face painful burns. Your body and soul took a tremendous beating. But when you reached your goal, your experience of the place was literally breathtaking and filled you with an amazement you had never felt before. It was a long, difficult, and costly journey for an experience that very few people can ever have—or even imagine. What an amazing memory you have to carry with you for the rest of your life. But it was a once-in-a-lifetime event, and you can't go back. That realization does not diminish the amazing things you experienced. In fact, it helps to put them in perspective—the immense physical effort and financial cost to get there remind you that this is a place not meant for humans to see. That makes the memory that much more precious—the realization that you saw the unseeable. You remember the amazement you felt, and you hold on to the beautiful memories, but you also know that you can never go back.

Crystal sex is like this amazing journey. Acknowledge the powerful, amazing pleasure you felt, costly in so many ways, to experience something that felt so amazing because the human brain was *never* meant to feel that. Unlike most people in this world, you were able to experience it and have incredible memories. *But you can never go back.* This is an important admission you need to make to yourself, because any hidden fantasy that one day you will have crystal sex again is a seed that can grow into an uncontrollable craving and a relapse.

When you are just starting to quit crystal, if sex is a significant trigger for you, then you may want to hold off on having sex for a while. This does not mean that you will never have sex again. Just for now give yourself a chance to work on basic recovery skills before you have sex again. Try for a month and see how well you do. It may take several months before you feel ready to tackle sex without crystal and feel safe that it will not lead to a relapse. Many people in CMA feel that if you are not currently in a relationship, it's best to try to stay away from sex for an entire year. For people who used to have frequent binges of crystal sex, who spent every weekend getting high while searching the Internet for sex, or who regularly used and did some other sexual activity, making a commitment of no sex for a year helps them to break those other habits that go along with crystal, which on their own can be addictive. Since sex is such a powerful trigger, those people may do better working on staying sober, learning relapse prevention skills, and practicing their ability to resist smaller urges before moving up to the challenge of sex, which will be tough, but eventually possible, and definitely enjoyable.

If one year sounds too long to you, set a shorter time limit that sounds tolerable for you, and see how you feel. At the end of that time, if you survived it and you think you would benefit from a little more time, then you can choose to wait a little longer. It is a good idea to give yourself a break, but set your time limit in bite sizes that you can swallow.

WHY REGULAR SEX SEEMS SO POINTLESS

DURING INITIAL SOBRIETY, sex just doesn't feel as good as it was when you did it with crystal. It's not just that everything in life is dull—sex in particular has lost its luster. The physiological reason is that after so much repeated and intense depletion of dopamine from the brain-reward circuit, the fibers in this pathway, which are associated with pleasure during sex, are damaged. Trying to stimulate the circuit again with sex just doesn't create the same charge it used to. This is true, not just for sex, but for many other activities that used to give you pleasure. Most of these things will improve over time. Your brain will gradually replenish its stores of dopamine, and some of those particular brain cells may recover, though unfortunately, some of the damage may be permanent. Lack of pleasure is worst right after stopping crystal. However, by one to two weeks, a good degree of your ability to feel pleasure should return as your dopamine stores are refilled. Recovery from damage to your brain cells, however, could take months to years.

Even after the initial crash, when most things in life feel better, sex still may seem empty. While this may be due in part to the neurological explanation described above, much of the difficulty is that, in comparison to sex on crystal, even imagining regular sex seems so dull. Figure 19-1 shows a scale of sexual pleasure experienced at different points in your life, from before your first sexual experience, through the time you were using crystal, and all the way to the time you are long into sobriety. The shaded area represents the normal range of pleasure that your brain experiences from different activities in life. Zero reflects no pleasure, and 10 is the highest pleasure that you normally feel, what should be *extremely* satisfying, such as having an orgasm.

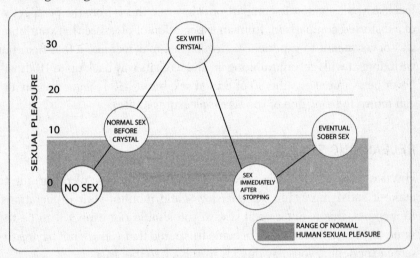

Figure 19-1. Scale of Sexual Pleasure

Think back to the *first* orgasm you ever experienced, whether you were masturbating or having sex with another person. It was so new and intense that it was probably off the pleasure scale compared to anything you had previous experienced, probably scoring a 15—off the charts if your normal pleasure scale is 0 to 10. That is why you very likely wanted to have an orgasm again. After repeating sex several times, it stopped feeling so new, but it remains extremely enjoyable, remaining at the top of your normal scale of pleasure, scoring your maximum of 10.

The first time that you had sex on crystal is similar to the first time you ever experienced an orgasm—so high that it is off the chart again. However, it is likely much higher than 15 because it is a physiological state that your brain could never reach on its own. On your scale of 0 to 10, sex on crystal would score a phenomenal 30—way off the charts. Looking at your previous experiences of sober sex, what seemed completely satisfying as a 10 now appears so low in comparison that it is like looking at a 0—bleak and empty. If it is so lackluster and boring, why would you want to do it again? Nonetheless, the drive to have sex will eventually return because it is a part of the brain-reward circuit. Almost inevitably, if sex became closely tied to crystal for you, sex will become a strong trigger for crystal because regular sex will likely not satisfy your sexual appetite at first. After repeated experiences of intense sex with crystal, the first several attempts at sober sex may feel like a pale shadow in comparison. However, this is from the perspective of a distorted comparison, from an expectation of pleasure that your brain was never meant to experience. Regular sex may feel like a 0 at first, but with time, it will feel enjoyable again and work its way back up to 10. It will never be as intense as the 30 of crystal sex, but it *will* feel good again and can return to being one of your great pleasures in life.

RELEARNING SEX

HAVING SEX AGAIN—*sober sex*—may require a process of relearning to make it satisfying again. Take it slowly and monitor your expectations. Remember, this is not crystal sex, so you should not expect it to be the same. If you rush yourself or become frustrated that you are not having the same experience, you may quickly turn back to the drug.

When you have sex, it is important not to have it in the same settings or situations in which you had crystal sex. You need to have different environmental cues, so that you do not trigger strong urges to use again. Stay clear of sex clubs, sex parties, telephone sex lines, Internet sex sites, any other places and activities that remind you of meth, or places where you know people are likely using it. Unless it is with your partner, do *not* have sex with people with whom you used to have crystal sex. Remove as many reminders of crystal sex from your life as you can. Even though you are not a virgin, imagine yourself starting something new and fresh. Detach yourself from *all* your older associations to sex that were in any way associated with crystal.

When first starting to have sex again, try to have it with someone who is not a random sex-only hookup. Set a rule of not having sex the first two times you meet someone, so you can get to know the other person and hopefully form a connection even before sex. Then when it's time to have sex, *take your time and go slowly*. Do not jump into the sex aggressively like a tiger pouncing on its prey—that is too much like the aggressive aspect of crystal sex, and you are exploring something different this time. Also, if you start the sexual encounter as you normally would with crystal sex, you start setting up expectations that it will feel like crystal sex. But it can't. Doing this sets yourself up for disappointment and frustration, and creates a trigger to go back to crystal.

For the relearning process, think of this as completely different activity. Focus on every little physical sensation: appreciate the feeling of holding the other person's hands and take in the sensation of skin rubbing against skin on the rest of the body. Wrap your arms around each other and gently hold each other, or if it feels good, enjoy a close and tight squeeze. How does it feel?

If you are both big kissers, don't just dive in as if you're fishing for pearls with your tongue in someone's throat—take your time and appreciate the the light touch of someone's lips against your own, or even the feeling of someone being so close that you feel the other person's warm breath against your lips or face, even before your lips ever touch. Again, go slowly, and take in what ever warm or happy emotions you may be feeling along the way. These are all the more intimate aspects of sex that trigger parts of your brain outside of the brain-reward circuit. They are more related to the parts that are activated by "connection" and "personal meaning," which have been found to be most closely associated with happiness. They are often forgotten or thrown by the wayside during the aggression of crystal sex, as the behaviors related to the brain-reward pathway crowd out most other things. Many people who have forgotten about the intense pleasure from the other parts of sex now realize that while sober sex will not be the same as crystal sex, it is not just a pale, weaker version—it is something different that has its own values that crystal sex will never have.

The first couple of times you have intimate physical contact with another person, restrict yourself to nongenital contact, even if you want to go further. Fully explore the intimacy and let the natural desire for sex build. You may find that you are much better able to feel an emotional pleasure that you may have been missing with crystal.

Many believe that crystal helped them feel "connected" to others when they had been feeling isolated. However, this is an *illusion*. While you may have been *physically* connected to someone while having wild, aggressive sex, it was the meth and the sex that you were really *emotionally* connected to, not the person, who could have been almost anybody. Consider how crystal was able to make almost anyone seem appealing, including people that you ordinarily would never have considered having sex with. Now you have the opportunity to experience a genuine connection to another person, and this is a wonderful feeling that crystal is not able to give you. Sober sex will begin to have its own positive associations, distinct from your memories of sex on crystal. However, be cautious. While relearning sober sex, if you slip and start to incorporate drugs into your sexual routine again, you are just contaminating your meth-free world with associations to meth and making the possibility of relearning satisfying sober sex more difficult.

When you are comfortable and enjoying the intimacy of sex without drugs, you can start to incorporate other things into your sexual activity to make it more exciting. Communicate with your partner about what feels good, or ask what your partner wants. Try role playing. Experiment and have fun. However, as much as possible, avoid activities that explicitly remind you of crystal sex.

While you will always have memories of sex on crystal, the desperate need to have it will gradually become less intense. Memories may return in flashes, but the flashes will become briefer and less frequent if you do not succumb to them by relapsing. Sex will eventually become the wonderful thing in your life that it had been before.

A SPECIAL NOTE FOR PEOPLE WITH SEXUAL COMPULSION/ADDICTION

PEOPLE WHO HAVE sexual compulsions and addictions likely had problems with sex even before crystal, though the drug can exacerbate the problem. These people should seek additional counseling to specifically address sexual compulsions, in addition to treatment for crystal addiction. Unless these compulsions are addressed, it will be much more difficult to break the associations of crystal and sex, because the compulsive aspect of this kind of sex is neurophysiologically tied to the pathways stimulated by crystal. You may need to address sex on a much slower time frame when trying to reintegrate it into your life.

One aspect of sex that is discussed above, the intimacy aspect, takes away the clandestine, secretive, and forbidden aspects of sex that is often part of the high in sexually compulsive behavior. Some psychologists theorize that, for sex addicts, the compulsion to have so much sex is an unconscious reaction against another unconscious force—the "superego" or conscience telling you that sex is bad. By going slowly with one partner and exploring intimacy and deep connection, you may be able to experience the sex not as something bad but as something beautiful, and this may lessen the desire to pursue sex compulsively. However, you should work with a specialist on this coaddiction to make sure you can keep it in control.

SPECIAL TOPICS

Topics are presented here for individuals with specific concerns in addition to the basic treatment program information presented. This is a small list of additional questions out of many that you may have about your own situation. I encourage you to think about any other questions and to be active in your search for answers. The process of doing and learning are important in your own recovery and in helping someone you love. More information is always helpful, being active in your pursuit of knowledge keeps the motivation alive, and any opportunity to understand the things that affect your life is important. After this section, there are resources listed in the appendices that may be able to assist you in pursing answers to more questions.

Topics:

- What if you slip and use crystal? Disaster and failure versus a learning opportunity and a step in the progress of recovery.
- Truly accepting yourself—are you just telling yourself "I'm a good person," or do you mean it?
- Crystal and HIV—how do these two completely different phenomena so intimately interact? How does each one affect the other? What you should know about crystal if you have HIV or want to stay HIV-negative.
- What do you do when someone you know has a problem with crystal?

20

WHAT IF YOU SLIP?
DOES IT MEAN FAILURE?

MOST PEOPLE WHO try to stop using crystal eventually "slip," meaning they eventually give in to temptation and use crystal again. A slip can be anything from accepting a single bump offered by a friend to having an entire weekend binge. The danger is that even a little slip can turn into a full relapse. What does it mean when you let your guard down and, after weeks, months, or years of working on staying clean, you use crystal again?

Before answering this question, it is important to remember that crystal addiction is a *chronic relapsing and remitting medical illness*. In everyday English, this means that it is a *lifelong* medical illness that can be *treated* but not *cured*. With treatment it gets better, though there will likely be periods when it worsens again. Similar common medical illnesses include high blood pressure and diabetes. Examining all three illnesses—addiction, high blood pressure, and diabetes—there is a remarkable similarity in the statistics of the three, most notably the rate of treatment adherence—actually sticking to the treatment recommendations; the percentage of people who improve, and the percentage who experience flare-ups in each of the different illnesses. The difficulty of sticking to treatment for diabetes and hypertension, as well as the high rate of flare-ups, suggests a high probability, that most meth addicts will slip at some time during their recovery.

In the past, people thought of staying clean versus slipping as equivalent to being cured or failing. However, according to the medical model, a slip is not failure. Few would call a diabetic whose blood sugar reading was high a failure, and while the person with diabetes, as well as friends and family, would be disappointed, the emotional reaction would not be as extreme as it is with a flare-up in drug addiction. Nonetheless, the profound disappointment in a slip is still a common response, and it creates a problematic effect, common enough that in addiction it has a specific label: the "abstinence violation effect." The expectation to stay clean "forever and always"—as opposed to the "just take each day as it comes" approach—creates a significant stress that can build up self-expectations to unrealistically high levels. If pressure is too intense, when a relapse occurs, the profound feeling of disappointment and the sense of hopelessness cause many people to give up. "I'm a failure at sobriety, so there is no point in trying anymore." There is a double danger to the abstinence violation effect: the motivated side of the crystal user that fights for sobriety loses hope, and the addicted side uses this as the perfect rationalization to keep using drugs and to forget about recovery. The addict in you now has free rein, since it has fooled the healthier part of you to surrender.

Take away the expectation that you will *never* slip. Lose the notion that a slip means failure. This *does not* mean you shouldn't hope that you will never slip. But getting rid of unrealistic expectations may alleviate much of the psychological pressure that can destroy your morale. Consider a twelve-year-old boy who dreams of becoming a basketball star. He loves to play on the courts every day after school. But if he expected to be perfect from the beginning and accepted no room for improvement, then after the first or second missed shot at the basket, he would give up, throw away his basketball, and never return to the court. But even this twelve-year-old-boy has more sense than to have such unrealistic and unforgiving expectations. To this kid who holds on to his dream of being a famous basketball player, missing the shot is disappointing, but it makes him want to practice even harder. *High hopes* are not the same as *impossible expectations*. Just focus on staying clean and sober in the present moment while you *hold on to the goal of a completely sober life.*

Accepting the possibility that you may slip does *not* mean that if you slip, you should keep using, because this is how the illness is supposed to be. The boy on the basketball court knows he will miss a lot of shots, but he never stops trying to make the next basket. In the medical model, a diabetic whose blood sugar has been rising wouldn't use this as a reason to gorge on more candy and toss away her insulin. Both the boy and the diabetic woman see their "slips" as signs that they need to work harder to improve. If you slip with crystal, or any other drug, it is appropriate to feel disappointed, but don't use it as an excuse to destroy your recovery. Move on and focus on how to get better.

If you have a therapist, a drug counselor, or a crystal relapse prevention group, work with them and use your experience as a learning opportunity. Examine what happened that led to the slip. Were there subtle signs that this was approaching? Had you been under more stress and how were you coping with it? Had you been spending more time in places or with people that were risky? Had you been keeping up with "the program," meaning going to CMA meetings, seeing your therapist, calling your sponsor, and so on? Had you been monitoring your stress level? How well were you managing it?

If you slip but don't try to learn from the experience, the likelihood of it happening again increases. Drug use may occur more frequently, and soon you may find yourself completely relapsing. On the other hand, if you use each slip as a learning opportunity, these setbacks can actually be steps that continue to lead you forward in your path to recovery. While slips are an expected part of addiction, if you continue to work hard at addressing them, they should gradually decrease in frequency and become easier to avoid.

21

YOU ARE WHO YOU ARE, AND THAT'S OKAY:
Acceptance—the Cornerstone of Staying Clean

> God grant me the serenity to accept the things I cannot change; the courage to change the things I can; and the wisdom to know the difference.
>
> —from *The Serenity Prayer*

ACCEPTANCE IS THE cornerstone of recovery. There are countless situations in which this acceptance applies, though in each situation it may be called something different, such as "surrendering," "letting go," "admitting," "accepting," "coming clean," and so on. In one form or another, they all boil down to acceptance, which is a powerful phenomenon.

In almost all religions, philosophies, and schools of thought, one of the ultimate goals is to bring peace and happiness, almost universally attained through some form of acceptance. Christianity teaches its believers to have *faith* in God and to accept his plan for his people. Buddhism teaches that suffering stems from ignorance and worldly desires, therefore *knowledge, mindfulness,* and *acceptance* of what you have will end suffering. The original teachings of Taoism espouse a natural order to the universe—harmony is achieved when people allow the world to be as it is, that is, to *accept their place in the universe and the natural flow of events*. In the West, cognitive psychologists reframe automatic thoughts that people have in situations that make them uncomfortable, finding ways to look at them that are more *acceptable.* Psychoanalysts believe that "anxiety," a psychoanalytic term that encompasses most negative emotional states, results when a person's desire (the id) conflicts with what the person feels is morally "good" (the superego). Psychoanalysis tries to help a person achieve inner peace by reducing this conflict and teaching the "self" (the ego) to find some way of *self-acceptance.*

It is remarkable that, from all parts of the world and from any point in history, almost every religion, philosophy, and psychological theory came to the same conclusion: acceptance, in some form, is fundamental to inner peace.

ACCEPTANCE THE TWELVE-STEP WAY

STEP ONE OF the Twelve Steps in CMA is to admit you are powerless over crystal. Most addicts believe that they are in good control of their use. Drug use at its core is an attempt to be in control. In particular, drug users try to control their emotions—for recreation or for relief of discomfort. "Feeling sad? I can *cheer up* with crystal. Going to a party where I'll be shy? I can *feel social* with crystal. The day feel boring? I can *spice it up* with crystal. Gradually you learn that if you keep using meth, as well as other drugs, you can control your feelings, which seems so much easier than tackling real-world problems that make you unhappy. Eventually you forget how to tolerate unpleasant feelings and to focus on fixing real problems, and troubles either continue or get worse.

What feels like an easy solution—using drugs—eventually gives you the narcissistic belief that you can handle almost anything—that is, as long as you have your drugs. And after so much experience fine-tuning your mood with drugs, it seems as if nobody else could possibly have as sophisticated an understanding of your mind and your brain as you. In time, it becomes almost impossible to hear anyone else's words as helpful.

As your illusion of control grows, the more crystal is actually gaining control over you. The drug you were using to manipulate your feelings is now manipulating you. In addition to signaling your primitive brain to use more of it, it has convinced you to ignore the rational part of your brain that would stop your drug use and try to approach problems without it. In addition, if you are a daily user, it has made you physically dependent, so you can't stop using it without feeling terrible. Though you had thought you were in control, meth now has you shackled in chains.

Accepting the fact that you are addicted to crystal and that you *do not* have control over it is one of the hardest admissions for an addict, because it contradicts the laws that govern this illusionary universe you live in. But *acceptance* is the starting point for recovery. Without it, as long as you don't wholeheartedly believe that crystal is controlling you, then *nothing* else in treatment will make any sense.

Accepting that one is "powerless" over crystal, and "surrendering" control, are extremely difficult, but once you accomplish these acts *and sincerely believe them*, you can feel surprisingly liberated. Keeping up the illusion that you are the "All-Powerful Controller," while the rational part of you watches your life fall apart from crystal, takes a lot of work. Letting go of the lie can actually be a tremendous relief.

ACCEPTANCE AND DEALING WITH FEELINGS

ONCE YOU HAVE accepted that you can't control all of your feelings, now you have to learn to tolerate them. As I mentioned on page 52, there is an AA saying "Hold your belly," which refers to an addict's tendency to complain ("Stop your bellyaching!") and to want a problem fixed immediately. It reminds people that they *can* get through unpleasant situations and encourages them to try to sit with the emotion and address problems without reaching for drugs. Feeling uncomfortable, angry, or sad will not kill you, though drugs may.

Not everything in life is pleasant, and not everything can be transformed into something wonderful. You may not be good at everything you do or get every job that you want for yourself. This is the *real* world, with both good and bad things. Adjust your expectations, accepting the reality that if some things don't turn out exactly as you had hoped, the world will not fall apart, and in most cases, you will be just fine. The world is *supposed* to be imperfect. If you understand and acknowledge the truth, rather than hide from it, you will be much better equipped to deal with it. With more realistic expectations, your disappointments will be fewer and easier to tolerate. Then coping with problems will be even easier and you may feel less compulsion to use drugs to hide from it.

WABI-SABI—MAKING AN ART OUT OF *NOT* BEING PERFECT

IN JAPAN THERE is an aesthetic called *wabi-sabi*, which developed from Zen Buddhism. It emphasizes an appreciation of the *imperfection* of all things in the world. People have tried various ways to translate the term—impermanence, transience, humility, asymmetry, imperfection—but none quite catch the essence. *Wabi-sabi* embraces the fact that nothing in nature is perfect, and this aspect of the natural world is not only accepted, it is revered. Japanese Zen Buddhism has even turned this into an art, prizing things that are imbalanced, rusted, or in some way reveal the decaying changes of time. The fleeting existence of all things—a flower, a person's youth, or life itself—makes them more precious. Therefore, it is all right that they are imperfect or that they will die because this is the natural way of the universe. If you can see your own imperfections as nature's wish, if you are able to accept not getting the job that you tried so hard to get, if you are able to accept that you may someday die—if you can let go of trying to control everything and making everything perfect, then the ups and downs of life come and go much more easily. With acceptance of the real world and more realistic expectations, you can live a happier life with more satisfaction.

ACCEPTANCE AND SAYING GOOD-BYE

THE PSYCHIATRIST ELISABETH Kübler-Ross described the stages of mourning as denial, anger, bargaining, depression, and acceptance. Remarkably, these are the same feelings that crystal addicts have when starting sobriety. Whether it is mourning the loss of a person or a drug, such as meth, these feelings are natural—*they are supposed to happen*. In recovery, it is expected that you will have these feelings—don't try to erase them by going back to crystal. Just like mourning the death of a loved one, it is important to experience these emotions in order to reach the final stage of acceptance that crystal is no longer a part of your life, and you will be able to feel peace.

22

CRYSTAL AND HIV:

How Do They Affect Each Other?

CRYSTAL AND HIV are intimately related, and they affect each other in countless ways: increasing your risk of getting HIV, treating the unhappiness of having HIV, worsening an HIV-positive person's general health, possibly making HIV even stronger, and injuring or destroying brain cells, especially when in combination. Much of this chapter refers to gay men or uses them in case examples because this is a group in which sex and crystal are often done together, and the prevalence of HIV is higher in this population. However, recent studies are beginning to show similar sexual patterns emerging among heterosexual people, so be aware that *the potential risks of crystal and HIV are the same for all users, gay or straight, male or female.*

As previously discussed, crystal stimulates neurological pathways that dramatically increase sexual desire and sexual activity, often with disregard for protecting oneself from STDs. This is even more frequently seen in communities that regularly use crystal in sexualized settings, such as gay circuit parties, sex clubs, and Internet sex sites. Although some recent statistics show that the rate of new HIV infections has finally leveled off

CRYSTAL AND HIV | 269

in the general population, the rate of new HIV infections continues to rise among the gay men, despite the fact that many, if not most, of these newly infected people already knew how to protect themselves.

Doctors working in the gay community have seen a frightening association between crystal use and HIV. The medical director of Callen-Lorde Community Health Center, for lesbian, gay, bisexual, and transgendered people in New York City, estimates that in 2004 approximately one-third of the clinic's patients who tested positive for HIV admitted that crystal was somehow related to their becoming infected. Other New York City physicians in private offices report similar statistics.

A joint study conducted by the University of California at San Francisco (UCSF) and the Centers for Disease Control (CDC) showed that of the gay men who reported using crystal meth between 2000 and 2001, 6.3 percent had been recently infected with HIV, compared to 2.3 percent of those who did not report using crystal. In other words, crystal almost tripled the chances of contracting HIV among these men. A study by Dr. Steven Shoptaw, an addiction specialist at UCLA, found that 61 percent of people seeking treatment for meth addiction at a particular clinic in California were also found to have HIV. Both in community experiences and in epidemiologic analyses, the medical community sees a *strong* connection between crystal and HIV.

WHY DOES CRYSTAL MAKE SEX SO MUCH MORE APPEALING?

WHAT IS IT about crystal that makes it so closely linked to HIV? Not only does it lower sexual inhibitions that prevent people from acting on their natural sexual urges, but for many people, it also drives the compulsion to have sex so intensely that concern for their health and protecting themselves from STDs, especially HIV, gets tossed out the window. Because sex and crystal stimulate the same brain-reward pathway, the compulsive drive to use crystal, against all logical sense, can also create a seemingly unstoppable drive to have sex.

Below is one man's description of his experiences of sex on crystal:

> Sex on crystal is amazing. There's nothing else like it. I feel like an animal on the hunt, and I'm determined to get my prey. I feel sexy and attractive, and the normal shy me is not really thinking about

whether I'm going to be rejected—I'm so focused on getting my next fuck. And it's easier to find sex because I'm so horny that I could fuck almost anyone, even someone I normally wouldn't think was attractive. When a trick comes over and I open the door, I almost don't even care what he looks like. He's just a piece of meat that I know I'm going to get to fuck. Before Viagra, crystal made me a total bottom because I couldn't get hard. I was okay with that because I could still get fucked for hours, and it was amazing. It was like I had this bottomless pit, this hunger to get fucked more. But once I started using Viagra with crystal, getting hard wasn't such a problem and I could top again—and fucking someone's ass, like I was attacking it, was so amazing, I could do it for hours—the feeling was *so* intense. Then when I'd finish with one person, I'd still be horny, so I'd move on to the next guy and continue my hunt [in a sex club or online].

In addition to sexual desire, other aspects of sex on crystal increase the risk of HIV transmission. Long periods of continuous rubbing against the lining of the anus, rectum, vagina, and mouth cause injury and damage to the mucosa (extremely delicate skin) lining these areas. Crystal also dries out the mucosa, making it even easier to damage from friction. Sex on meth is often physically aggressive, so penetration can be rough and forceful, causing even more cuts, tears, and abrasions. *Any* small break in the mucosa is an open door for HIV to enter the body and cause a new infection, and all of the conditions mentioned above increase the risk that HIV can infect someone by opening more doors for the virus to pass through. The risk of becoming infected with HIV is also higher for the person penetrating the partner, or the "top," because hours of continuous rubbing of the penis against *anything*–hand, anus, vagina, and so on—will create small cuts and abrasions on the surface. Without a condom to shield them, those small cuts are also entryways for HIV into your body.

As described by the crystal user above, the drive to have sex can be so overwhelming that it causes many people to disregard their usual precautions, because sex is their number one priority. The mind-blowing sex on meth feels so important, and even urgent, that everything else seems trivial: users ignore the need to rest, drink, or eat, let alone take the extra effort to use a condom. Many users already know the risks of HIV, but when they are having sex on crystal, any interference with sexual pleasure, such as decreased sensation with a condom, feels intolerable.

Crystal has been so clearly linked to the spread of HIV and other sexually transmitted diseases that a joint study by UCSF and the CDC clearly stated in its conclusion that to *successfully* contain the epidemic of HIV, methamphetamine use *must* be reduced,

IF YOU ALREADY HAVE HIV, HOW CAN CRYSTAL AFFECT YOU?

PEOPLE WHO ALREADY have HIV aren't concerned about getting it. However, there are still many ways that crystal can harm them, specifically with regard to their HIV infection. A significant issue is crystal's effect on the immune system in general, as well as its ability to fight the HIV that is already in the body. In studies of HIV-positive people, crystal use was associated with an increase in the amount of HIV in the blood and a decrease in **CD4 cells** (commonly called "T-cells," or specifically "helper T-cells," a type of white blood cell that is essential to the body's ability to fight infections). The reasons for these effects are not clear. Meth may affect HIV itself, it may affect the immune system, or it may affect people's ability to stick to their regimen of HIV medications.

Numerous studies have consistently shown that when people are high on crystal, they are much more likely to miss taking their HIV medications. Depending on which medications are prescribed, people must stick closely to their regimen—at least 95 to 98 percent of the time—to keep HIV under control and to prevent it from becoming resistant to the medications. The difficulty in sticking to medication regimens is likely the *most* significant cause of worsening HIV levels and immune function in meth users who have HIV.

In *vitro* (test tube) studies of HIV living in cell cultures have shown that methamphetamine accelerates HIV replication five to fifteen times faster than the replication of HIV not exposed to the drug. Because viruses and cells in test tubes do not always act the way they would in the complex environment of living bodies, it is important to see how methamphetamine affects the virus in living animals (in vivo). Feline immunodeficiency virus (FIV) is a cat virus that behaves similarly to HIV but affects cats, and it is similar enough to HIV that it is frequently used as a model for how HIV might behave in the human body. Just as in the test tubes studies, the virus in FIV-positive cats given methamphetamine multiplied much more rapidly than in cats not given any drug. It likely has a similar effect in the human body. Both test tube and animal studies consistently show that crystal increases HIV replication. The implication is that the same is true for humans. One human study clearly showed that levels of HIV increased when people used crystal; however, those people also stopped taking their medications, so it is not possible to conclude that crystal itself increased HIV production..

CRYSTAL AND THE BODY'S IMMUNE SYSTEM

THE SCIENTIFIC COMMUNITY has long known that amphetamine, a weaker cousin of methamphetamine, impairs immune function, consistently demonstrated in both in vitro and in vivo studies. Further recent research specifically with methamphetamine has shown similar results, disrupting immune function in several ways.

An extremely significant effect of crystal is that it lowers the number of **CD8 cells** that circulate throughout the body. CD8 cells, a subtype of immune cell known as "killer T-cells," respond to chemical signals from CD4 cells ("helper T-cells") by multiplying and forming a strong army to attack invading infections. Killer T-cells are the first line of defense when a person is exposed to HIV. The strength of the immune system's initial response to the virus has a crucial impact on how the person being infected with HIV will fare in the future. Some scientists theorize that the stronger the initial CD8 response, the more effectively the body fights the initial HIV infection. The less overwhelmed the body is by the first infection, more of the immune system is preserved to fight infections and maintain good health for a longer period down the road.

Some scientists postulate that the strength of the CD8 response to the body's first exposure to HIV significantly affects the viral "set point" for that individual—the level where the virus temporarily remains after the initial infection. The lower the viral set point, the longer the time before HIV breaks from its quiet state, multiplying faster and faster and wreaking havoc. The less overwhelming the first attack by HIV, the better the immune system seems to be able to keep the virus in check. A strong initial CD8 response to the body's first exposure to HIV may result in a lower set point, and a longer period of good health. A weak CD8 response may have a higher viral set point, and HIV may progress to AIDS more quickly.

Using crystal when one is infected with HIV may result in serious health consequences down the line.

Methamphetamine also interferes with B lymphocyte function. B cells, a different type of immune cell, produce antibodies, one of the immune system's strongest weapons against viruses, bacteria, and other invading microorganisms. Methamphetamine blocks B-cells from responding to chemical signals that orchestrate an organized response against an infection. Normally, B cells respond to the correct signal by multiplying and producing antibodies to kill a foreign microorganism, but in the presence of meth, the B cell response is significantly lower..

Crystal disrupts the function of the immune system in many other ways, as well. For example, it is also associated with lower levels of chemicals that immune cells use to communicate with each other, such as interleukin-2 and gamma-interferon. It is also associated with an increase in tumor necrosis factor (TNF), a chemical that has been found to accelerate the progression of HIV. All of these derangements significantly prevent the immune system from functioning properly.

If you have HIV, you should *optimize* your immune function. Clearly, crystal does the exact opposite.

CRYSTAL, HIV, AND THE BRAIN

PREVIOUSLY I DISCUSSED in detail how crystal damages brain cells. Similarly, HIV is toxic to the brain. The combination of the two can result in even greater brain damage.

To review briefly, crystal damages or destroys cells in the **thalamus** (affecting numerous functions ranging from attentiveness to the perception of pain) and the **basal ganglia** (involved with movement, motivation, learning, and impulse control).

HIV affects similar parts of the brain, in particular the basal ganglia, as well as many other deep-brain structures located beneath the cerebral cortex. The proteins on the outer coating of the virus, especially Tat and gp120 proteins, are particularly toxic. These proteins indirectly affect neurons by destroying **astrocytes**, the supportive cells that protect, nourish, and assist the function of brain cells. Without astrocytes, many brain cells cannot function properly and many of them die. Similar to crystal, HIV significantly affects the basal ganglia, as well as other subcortical regions. The pattern of brain damage caused by both HIV and crystal is called "subcortical dementia," meaning that they damage deep-brain structures, unlike Alzheimer's disease, which affects the superficial cortex. Subcortical dementia is characterized by slow mental processing, impaired decision making, and difficulty performing complex mental tasks.

In animal studies using cats with FIV, as well as monkeys with simian immunodeficiency virus (SIV—thought to be the direct ancestor of HIV), methamphetamine caused a significant increase in viral replication, and this increase was even greater in the brain than in other areas of the body. In humans, the level of HIV in the brain can be as much as ten times greater than the level measured in the rest of the body. Therefore, people taking HIV medications who have "undetectable" levels of HIV in the blood may still have a significant amount of virus in the brain, and crystal use can make the HIV already there multiply even faster.

William F. Maragos and colleagues at the University of Kentucky conducted an experiment exposing one group of animals to crystal, another group to the Tat protein of HIV, and a third group to both crystal and Tat. Animals exposed to crystal showed an 8 percent reduction of dopamine function in the striatum. Those exposed to Tat protein showed a 7 percent reduction in dopamine function. Animals exposed to *both* crystal and Tat had a surprising 65 *percent* decrease in dopamine function. Brain function was measured one week after exposure to crystal and Tat, showing that these were effects that persisted after crystal exposure. Another animal study by Chapman and colleagues showed that brain damage in mice was notable even three weeks after exposure to meth.

The lesson here is that crystal and HIV each cause brain damage, and, in combination, the toxicity is extremely high and persists even after the drug is stopped.

CRYSTAL AND HIV MEDICATIONS

CRYSTAL, LIKE ANY other chemical that is put into the body, can interact with many medications, including those for HIV. Among the HIV meds, protease inhibitors are particularly dangerous to combine with meth, as are many other recreational drugs because they slow the ability of the liver to break down other chemicals, drugs, and medications. A notoriously potent protease inhibitor is ritonovir (Norvir). Its slowing effect has been used to boost the blood levels of other medications to make them more effective.

However, it can also allow drugs and medications to accumulate to toxic levels that can be deadly. At least one published case report attributed a death to the mixture of HIV medications and crystal. In this person, an *extremely* high level of meth was measured in the blood that would have been difficult to achieve by normal crystal use.

There are other non-HIV medications that can also inhibit the breakdown of crystal, including several psychiatric medications for depression and anxiety; cimetidine (Tagamet) for indigestion and peptic ulcer disease; quinidine, a heart medication; ketoconazole, an antifungus medication; and many others.

Crystal can have other dangerous interactions with medications. For example, in patients taking a certain kind of antidepressant called monoamine oxidase inhibitors (MAOIs), crystal can cause extreme high blood pressure that can lead to a stroke. Just as you should always ask your doctor if it is safe to combine over-the-counter cold medicine with your prescription medications, you need to find out if crystal is safe in combination, as well.

An important consideration: if your HIV medications are life saving and you find out that your medications are not safe with crystal, what is your reaction? If you even consider the possibility of stopping the life-saving medications so that you can take crystal, is that a strong enough indication of how much power crystal has over you? Why would you be willing to trade your life for a brief high?

CRYSTAL, HIV, AND OTHER PARTS OF THE BODY

CRYSTAL AFFECTS ALMOST every part of the body outside of the brain. It increases body temperature and can result in muscle breakdown, which in its severe form is called **rhabdomyolysis**. This is even more likely to happen when someone uses crystal on the dance floor, where he or she is continuously active and overheated, does not rest, and is dehydrated. These conditions increase the risk of rhabdomyolysis, which can potentially turn into an uncontrollable cascade of muscle breakdown. The muscle byproducts of rhabdomyolysis are toxic to the kidneys, and if they overwhelm the kidneys too quickly, kidney damage could turn into kidney failure.

Like all stimulants, crystal increases heart rate and blood pressure. Both of these changes make the heart work harder, trying to pump an adequate supply of blood to the entire body, including the blood vessels that nourish the heart itself. When the heart works harder, it requires more oxygen, which is carried in the blood that it pumps. For people with certain heart diseases, such as coronary artery disease (clogged arteries in the heart), crystal is particularly dangerous because there is *already* a problem delivering enough blood to their hearts under normal circumstances. Increasing the heart's need for more blood increases the likelihood of a heart attack.

People with HIV who are taking an HIV cocktail (**highly active antiretroviral treatment,** or **HAART**) also are at risk for heart problems because these medications, especially the protease inhibitors, can cause astronomical increases in cholesterol and triglyceride levels. These are associated with clogged arteries, heart attacks, and strokes. For people taking HAART, there is a 5 percent cumulative annual risk of having some heart-related illness. This means that *each* year you continue to take your HAART regimen, there is an *additional* 5 percent risk of heart disease. Over five years, that is a 25 percent increase in risk. HAART is life saving and has changed the way that HIV is seen today. However, its price is potential toxicity—in this example to the heart—and people taking HAART still need to be careful about their health.

Heart disease caused by HIV medications may never be recognized until an actual heart attack or stroke occurs. Therefore, if you are taking HAART, you may not even realize that you have some heart disease. For you, using crystal is particularly risky. This is not just a theory—unfortunately, there have been several cases of young HIV-positive men who had heart attacks while using crystal. There are likely many cases of small heart attacks that are never reported or documented. Most meth users are younger than the elderly people that we associate with heart attacks, so some meth users who experience mild chest pain may not even consider the possibility that they are having a heart attack—they may let it pass without giving it a second thought. Some of my crystal-addicted patients have experienced chest pains and *did* consider the possibility that they were having heart attacks, but they did not go to the ER because they feared others would learn that they used the drug. Their addiction was so strong that keeping their crystal use a secret was more important than protecting their life. Fortunately, they did not die. But they could have.

23

WHAT DO YOU DO
IF SOMEONE YOU KNOW
HAS A PROBLEM WITH CRYSTAL?

THIS CHAPTER IS for people who know someone who is addicted to crystal: a friend, a
family member, a partner, a spouse, a coworker, or anyone else in your life
who you think is hooked on meth. You may be worried, sad, frustrated with,
or even exasperated by this person and the addict he or she has become.
The prospect of dealing with someone so controlled by a drug may seem
impossible because his or her behavior is so stubborn and resistant to change.
Meanwhile, you are left feeling powerless to help as you watch the addiction
destroy your loved one. Each person who has an addiction is different and
should be approached according to his or her unique situation. This chapter
is intended to be a general guide to help you structure your own approach,
to provide a basic framework to your plan so that you can feel that there is a
logical rationale to whatever your do. Keep in mind that there are many ways
of dealing effectively with addicts, and this chapter discusses only some of the
many possible strategies to consider.

Before thinking about what to say to an addict, it is important to understand what he or she is experiencing as thoroughly as you can without

actually using the drug yourself. Read the chapters in parts 1 and 2 to learn as much as you can about crystal—what it is, how it works, and how it makes people feel, both the good and the bad. Also read the chapters that define addiction and see if this reflects what you see in the person who concerns you.

Armed with that knowledge, if you see true addiction, this chapter may offer you some useful guidance on how to deal with the addicted person in your life.

ADDICTED FRIENDS OR FAMILY MEMBERS

IF YOU ARE dealing with addiction in someone particularly close to you, the thought of confronting that person can be daunting because you may be afraid of pushing him or her away. At the same time, if you do *nothing* while the addiction continues, you are much more likely to lose that person from your life, and worse yet, he or she could even die as a result of the drug. If the addict is someone you care about, stepping in to help is one of the best things you can do, even if it means being rejected.

To lay the groundwork, I hope you have read the other chapters mentioned above and understand that both biological and psychological processes are dictating the behavior of your loved one. He or she did not become addicted because he or she is stupid, weak, or bad. Something pleasurable or psychologically *helpful* about crystal enticed the person to start using crystal, and that helpful quality, together with its strong neurophysiological basis, keeps this person continuing use it, despite all of the obvious problems that you see it has caused. Try to find out what those positive things, are so that you can understand why it is so difficult to quit meth.

Think back to what your loved one was like before crystal and look at what you see now. If there is a dramatic difference, you can see the power of meth on the human mind and body. The person that you knew before crystal took hold is still in there somewhere. However, many of the behaviors and moods you see—lying, hiding, withdrawing, moodiness, irritability, paranoia, rageful outbursts, depression, and so on—are a result of crystal highs, crashes, and cravings. Most of these behaviors are resolved when addicts become sober, though addiction also causes some changes in character that are difficult to change back.

Recognizing the behaviors and moods caused by crystal addiction is essential to give you clearer vision when you observe them. When you confront your loved one, if you meet angry resistance, you can better see what behaviors and words are symptoms of the addiction, which may help you not to take angry words too personally. If a friend broke his leg, would you expect him to accompany you on a mountain hike? Of course not. You consider his limitations based on what he has to work with—a bum leg. Similarly, addicts are working with a chemically altered mood, a physiologically based compulsion to continue using, and a neurologically impaired ability to make judgments. As with the friend with the broken leg, you cannot expect the person to react in the most rational way when told to quit. If you make your expectation more realistic, you can be less emotionally vulnerable if your loved one responds to your goodwill with anger and denial. You may feel less of the bite of angry personal attacks against you, and this may allow you to feel more compassion than frustration.

How to Discuss the Problem

There are several ways to tell a loved one that you are concerned about his or her crystal use: a private one-on-one conversation, a group discussion with other friends or family members, or the traditional intervention. There is no one single right way to do it. You may need to experiment with different tactics. I usually prefer to test the waters with a one-on-one talk because it is less intense and confrontational. The response can give you an idea of how receptive or resistant the person is. If a one-on-one conversation accomplishes little, at least it has given you some information about how much resistance you are working against. This will help you decide how much intensity you need for the next step—bringing in a crucial and influential person, having a group conversation, or cranking up the heat to a group confrontation or all the way up to a fully orchestrated intervention in which family and friends make prepared statements and the discussion is facilitated by an experienced leader. For an intervention, a predetermined rehabilitation program is often arranged so that if the person agrees to treatment for his or her addiction, the process can start immediately, before he or she has a change of heart.

When to Have the Talk

Choosing the right time to talk can have a significant impact on how receptive your loved one is to your words. When addicts are high on crystal or any other substance, this is obviously not the right time. If they have not used crystal for several weeks, they may be in a more rational state. However, they may also be feeling so well because the pain of the crash has waned and denial is easy. Because they feel all right at the moment, they can easily rationalize their behavior. Consider talking to them during a crash. They may be feeling tired, depressed, anxious, or generally miserable. At that particular moment they may actually welcome an offer for help because they feel so distressed and vulnerable. Take advantage of the times when they are so aware of the bad effects of crystal that they are impossible to deny. On the other hand, they may be feeling so tired and irritable that they crave more crystal to help themselves feel better. Being so focused on that, they will not be at all receptive to outsiders' comments. Perhaps the *best* time to talk is soon after the crash, when they feel better enough to have a conversation, but have the recent memory of an unpleasant crash still very fresh in their minds. During that particular period, addicts may be the most motivated to stop using drugs. Because motivation and insight change constantly, be on the lookout for a good window of opportunity.

Before you have your talk, be prepared. Make a list of all the things you want to cover and how you are going to say them, choosing wording that is honest about your feelings but nonjudgmental. You know the situation will be uncomfortable for both of you, and strong emotional reactions can throw you off guard. A defensive person may try to engage you in circular, illogical arguments, and you will quickly find yourself derailed from your original plan. Keep yourself close to your framework and use a mental script (or a written script—write it as if it were a letter, and it won't sound so unnatural if you have to read your own words) that will allow you to emotionally step back and stay focused on your point.

What to Discuss

Start the conversation with positive comments, for example, "I love you very much," or "You are one of the most important people in my life, and our friendship means so much to me." Use your first comment to establish a supportive tone for the rest of the conversation. If you begin with criticism or even a sympathetic comment with negative overtones, such as "I'm worried about you," the conversation has already become confrontational, and your loved one will *immediately* take a defensive position, shutting his or her ears to whatever discussion follows. A positive statement at the beginning reminds *both* of you why you are having this talk—because this person matters dearly to you, and vice versa. Hopefully a loving and supportive start will soften up the person's defensive reactions a little, and if he or she becomes hostile and combative, think of your first statement to remind yourself that you are having this conversation because you care, not because you are angry and want to cause someone else emotional pain. Keep reminding yourself about this point so that you can step back and try not to become engaged in heated, emotional arguments.

Identify recent behaviors that you have seen or that are factually indisputable. For example, your friend did not show up to meet you for dinner; she has been missing days of work every week; he has admitted to having unprotected sex and has contracted several sexually transmitted diseases. The more specific you can be, the less room you leave for argument or denial.

Frame these behaviors as concerns that you have for someone you very much care for, not as accusations. Monitor your language and tone of voice—speak slowly, and keep your volume low and the pitch of your voice from getting higher and tighter. This will prevent you from sounding critical or attacking and will reduce the likelihood of a defensive reaction. Remain calm and caring.

Remind your loved one about his or her *own* goals and desires in life: friends, family, career, education, or whatever else he or she considers important. Use these as the measuring sticks for explaining how well or badly the addict has been doing while under the influence of crystal. Avoid describing any problems in terms of *your* own hopes or disappointments; otherwise, the person will only become more convinced that you do not understand or care at all. Your loved one will try to believe, and try to convince you, that you are only interested in yourself. Resist the urge to feel guilty or to question your own motives. You already know that you are trying to show your loved one his or her own problems, not yours.

Have list of recommendations prepared—possibilities include working with a drug counselor; checking out local twelve-step meetings; joining a non–twelve-step support group about addiction; reading a book, such as this one, to learn more about crystal; or going to rehab. Do not leave a discussion about problems without any possible solutions, otherwise it will truly feel like criticism and can leave the person feeling hopeless.

Your addicted friend or family member may not immediately accept your message that there is a problem. He or she may still be in too much denial or may be feeling so defensive that it may take a little time alone to digest your comments. At the very least, having the conversation shows the person that you are available as a caring support around the issue of crystal addiction, and that if he or she ever wants to address the addiction, there are specific ways to get help.

Do Not Get Emotional

Confronting loved ones about their addictions is extremely difficult, but being on the receiving end of a confrontation is even harder. Expect that your friend or relative will be defensive, even angry, and more than likely he or she will argue and try to oppose everything you say. The person may retaliate by trying to provoke the same angry or hurt feelings in you. Remind yourself that this is part of the addiction, and if you start feeling anger well up, stop talking, take a deep breath, and go back to the discussion framework that you prepared. If you let yourself become angry, the discussion changes from a rational discussion to an emotional battle. Then you give the person good reason not to listen to you, and the natural reaction in a fight is to push against anything thrown out by the opponent. Instead, remain calm and compassionate.

What to Expect

Friends and relatives have all sorts of reactions to "the talk." Some may be able to listen and feel grateful for your support. Unfortunately, most people are not so receptive. Despite your best efforts to keep the discussion from turning into an argument, you will usually encounter some defensiveness and denial. However, that does not mean that the person did not hear you. If you see a severe problem, more than likely he or she sees it, too. Even when the person is able to admit to some of the points you bring up, do not expect to end your discussion in total agreement. Knowing that complete agreement is not the goal will help you to back off at the right time and not feel so frustrated. When you end the discussion, accept that there may still be disagreement between you, mentally step back, let the person know that you are still there for support, and leave the person to think about the things you have discussed. The conversation may take place several times in a variety of ways. But keep giving a consistent message: you care about this person, he or she has a problem, and you think he or she can get better.

After the Talk, What Else?

Now that you have voiced your concern, follow though with what you said. Do not disappear, but remain present as a support. If the person decides to take the plunge and quit meth, he or she will be going through an arduous period of physical, emotional, and mental changes. Your loved one may need your help now, more than ever, to get through the depression, moodiness, and agonizing cravings of quitting.

Spend time together and show how important it is to you that this person is trying to clean up, and engage in activities that do not involve drugs or alcohol. Remind each other what your interpersonal bond is really about and enjoy each other's company in a meaningful way. You are literally competing with crystal, which may have become your loved one's new "best friend." But the friendships are different—one is chemical, compulsive, destructive, and out of control, while your is deep, meaningful, emotional, and supportive. You hope that at some point the person will see this.

When you spend time together, do not constantly focus on drugs, always monitoring the other person's behavior and asking what he or she has been doing. The person may feel overly scrutinized, self-conscious, or embarrassed, especially right after being confronted. Allow a little breathing room after your discussion. But if you detect new problems or a downward spiral into the old, have another talk.

Above all else, if you yourself do drugs, do not use crystal or other drugs in front of the person you are trying to help. How can he or she take you seriously if *you* are not able to stop using drugs? Model healthy, drug-free behavior and demonstrate that you can enjoy yourselves without drugs. Also, keep in mind that the even the sight of anything associated with drugs can trigger physiological reactions in the brain that cause intense craving. Why would you put this person through that agony? Using drugs in front of recovering addicts is disrespectful of their efforts to stay clean, and it is downright cruel. Would you insist that a friend with severe asthma visit your grandmother and her twenty cats? Don't do things that will increase your loved one's risk of relapsing, and give him or her great respect for working so hard at sobriety.

If your friend or family member has been successful at staying away from drugs, give positive reinforcement and acknowledge that he or she is doing a great job, but do not be patronizing. Overcoming crystal addiction is truly a tremendous feat. Do not underestimate the difficulty, and consider yourself lucky if you never have to face such a challenge. Mean it when you say, "Wow, it's been three weeks without any crystal and you're doing great!"

Setting Limits

If your loved one is not able to stop using crystal, set some limits as to what you will tolerate. A buddy who never shows up, lies, or asks for money and never pays it back can become an annoyance. A sister who constantly calls up for support because she fears she caught another STD after another story of unprotected sex on crystal can become tiresome, if not exhausting. You may start to feel annoyance, resentment, and even dread building up whenever you hear the person's voice, knowing that regardless of your warnings about crystal and risky sexual behavior, nothing ever changes. Your reaction is a sign that you are burning out. Set some limits to protect yourself and your relationship.

On the other hand, instead of feeling irritated by such behaviors, some people feel the opposite—concerned and overprotective. This can be problematic if it leads you to ignore dangerous warning signs, cover up for your loved one when he or she misses appointments or work, or help to pay rent or other bills because money is always spent on crystal instead. This type of behavior is called "enabling." You may do it out of love and concern, but in the end, it allows the addict to continue using drugs even longer because he or she never has to face the difficult consequences. If you stop making excuses for your loved one, he or she may get into trouble at work or even get fired. Without your financial assistance, he or she may get evicted and become homeless. As horrible as it sounds to let this happen to someone you care about, it may take just such a dramatic loss to break the illusion that crystal creates—that everything will be all right, as long as there is more crystal.

Think about what your limits are. What can you tolerate, and which of your behaviors may be enabling? Carefully decide what you believe is helpful support versus what will fuel the addiction. Expect that your loved one will try to put a lot of emotional pressure on you and make you feel guilty for bailing him or her out of trouble. Being prepared with your limits will let you withstand the emotional pressure and help you to feel confident that the help you give—or refuse to give—is for a good reason. For example, you may offer to be available to your friend at any time, day or night, for emotional support; however, you will not lend any money, and you will not participate in any activities with this person that may involve drugs.

After you decide what your limits are, explain them to your loved one making the terms as explicit and concrete as possible, with no room for misinterpretation, loopholes, or excuses. Some examples of clearly defined limits are: "I will not lend you any money," or "We will not engage in any activities where drugs may be around, and if drugs are there, I will leave." Addicts, especially when they are desperate, can be excellent lawyers, relentlessly arguing almost any case. "But you said that if I needed money for food . . ." "This time is different—I'm sick and I need to go to the doctor." Make your limits so clear that there is no question. You are never the only option for an addict. Even in worst-case scenarios, there is almost always another option: for the sick, there is the emergency room; for the homeless, there are shelters. Sometimes it takes extremes such as these to make addicts understand how much their lives have changed because of crystal.

Whatever limits you set for yourself, stick to them. Be gentle and caring, but be firm. If your addicted son tries to manipulate you with guilt, find other ways to help without overstepping your limits. If your addicted friend is sick but has no insurance and can't afford medical care, take her to the free city clinic or offer to help take her to the nearest Medicaid office, where she can apply for help herself. These are not glamorous options, but this is exactly what your loved one needs to see. Addicts needs to face up to just how ugly things have really become. Only then will they realize that they need to change.

Do not exceed your limits, thinking, "Just this once, when he really needs my help." Doing so may actually worsen the situation. Consider the classic behavioral science experiment with mice. Mice can be trained to hit a lever by pairing it with a reward, such as receiving a pellet of food. If they receive food after hitting the lever five times, they continue to hit the lever in order to get more food. If food pellets are no longer delivered, the mouse keeps trying, but after numerous unsuccessful attempts, the mouse eventually gives up and forgets about the lever. The behavior is "extinguished." If, however, instead of *completely* stopping the food supply, you allow some food pellets to fall at random times when the lever is pushed, the mouse will continue pushing the lever. This is called "intermittent positive reinforcement." Randomly giving the food pellet actually makes the mouse continue to push the lever even more tenaciously than if you were giving it at a predictable rate. The mouse does not know when the food will come, but he knows that if he diligently keeps pushing the lever, food will eventually come.

The exact same phenomenon occurs in humans. If you set a limit but on rare, "extreme" occasions, you ignore your restrictions "because it was a special situation," the addict then learns that, if he or she is persistent enough, you will eventually cave in and do what he or she wants. Then the limits become meaningless. Rather than understand your limits as an important part of recovery, the addict will focus on how to get you to exceed your limits again.

What Happens If the Person Relapses?

Once someone decides to stop crystal, no matter how well he or she does in recovery, relapse is always a possibility. In fact, it is likely that it will eventually happen. If someone starting out in recovery starts using crystal again, do not despair or lose hope. Remember that addiction is a chronic relapsing and remitting disease, meaning that once people have it, they have it forever—there will be stable periods, but there may also be flare-ups. When a woman with hypertension has been able to control her blood pressure for years, but her blood pressure spikes, is she a failure? No—it's the nature of the illness. She needs to try to get it back under control and change or intensify her treatment.. For friends and family, this model is helpful because it provides more realistic expectations and helps decrease frustration and burnout.

In crystal addiction, some relapses are expected, and a few fallbacks, some might argue, may be help to show how "powerless" the addict is, despite the most sincere desire and efforts to stop. Instead of feeling frustration and despair, try to help the addict use the initial relapses as learning opportunities.

Get Support

You should not go through the experience of dealing with an addicted family member or friend alone. Some resources of support include Al-Anon meetings (support groups specifically for friends and family of addicts) and psychotherapists experienced with addiction issues. Do not isolate yourself. Talk to people about what you are going through. Al-Anon can be particularly helpful because it offers peer support from other people in situations similar to yours, and it teaches proper limit setting and how to recognize unintentional enabling behavior. At Al-Anon meetings, you can check in with others when you are feeling uncertain or doubtful about whether you are being too strict or too lax, and you can reinvigorate your motivation when you feel emotionally depleted. Most important, Al-Anon helps you accept the fact that there is only so much that you can do. You can test your limits by sharing them in the meetings, and you will feel more comfortable with what you do—and what you refuse to do—in order to help the addicted person.

When to Pull Back

When is enough enough? If violence or abuse is ever involved, pull out. Your own safety comes first. If you find that you cannot stick to limits that you set, or if your friend or relative continues to push you, manipulate you, or treat you badly, and all attempts to change this have failed, then your relationship with this person may have turned completely toxic. If continuing your present relationship has not been productive but instead it has been destructive to you personally and to the relationship itself, then it may be time to pull back. Pulling back does not mean giving up on the addict, though he or she may experience it as such. It means putting an end to a way of interacting that is harmful to both of you. If you have questions about whether you have reached this point, ask other people in your support network, especially other people who have been in the same situation as you, or discuss your situation with an addiction specialist.

If you decide to pull away, you are not deserting your loved one. To make this clear, explain exactly what you are doing: "I'm sorry, but I can't spend time with you anymore. It seems like no matter what we plan, you keep disappearing because you're getting high, or it seems like you're always asking me for money. Nothing has really changed, and I won't go on like this. You are my friend (or brother/whatever), and I am here for you if you want to get better from this addiction. But I've tried everything I can to help you, and nothing has worked. So you need to change in order to be in my life again."

It sounds strong, and it feels harsh, but sometimes it must be done. A 45-year-old woman told be about her struggles with her twenty-two-year-old son, who was a crystal addict. The mother and son truly loved each other. However, the son's addiction was so strong that no matter what limits the mother put on his interactions with him, her son found ways to get around them. When she invited her son over for dinner, she later discovered he had stolen some of her expensive possessions to sell for crystal. Once her son took her car without permission. Despite the love that the mother and son felt for each other, the addiction was so strong that the son betrayed his mother repeatedly to feed his need for crystal. As difficult as it was, the woman had to sever ties with her son. She realized that unless she stopped enabling him, he would never find his way out of his addiction. Losing this precious relationship was one of the major negative consequences that the addicted son needed to experience. Eventually, he came to see that crystal cost him more than money—it almost cost him one of the most important people in his life. Two years later the son decided to go to rehab. Now he is working seriously on recovery and he has reestablished contact with his mother.

ADDICTED PARTNERS, SPOUSES, AND SIGNIFICANT OTHERS

IF THE CRYSTAL addict in your life is not just a friend or relative but is your partner (life companion, spouse, boyfriend or girlfriend, domestic partner, or however you describe the person with whom you share your life), everything mentioned above applies, though your situation could be much more complicated. If you live together, you are much more emotionally interdependent, and you may be financially intertwined with joint bank accounts and property. For all these reasons and more, your behavior and emotional reactions have a greater impact on each other.

Is your partner lying to you, using up the money in your joint account, stealing from you, or cheating on you? If you have a sexually open relationship, is your partner having more sex outside the relationship? Is your partner having unprotected sex with others and potentially exposing you to STDs? Is your partner getting high and forcing you to have sex when you don't want to or in ways that are so aggressive that you don't enjoy it?

With all these questions running through your mind, do you feel you can trust this person with whom you share everything? You may feel angry, frustrated, or cheated. If your partner really cared about you, how could he or she act with such blatant disregard for you? And if you cannot trust your partner, why should you even stay together as a couple? These are some of the heart-wrenching questions that partners of crystal addicts struggle with.

To make sense of this confusing situation, keep in mind that some of the behavior you are seeing is likely the addiction rather than the person you used to know and love. Ask yourself if your partner was like this before using crystal. Try to distinguish the difficulties in your relationship from the symptoms of crystal addiction. If some of the behavior is clearly due to drug use, withdrawal, or uncontrollable craving, then the enemy may be the addiction, though it seems as if it's your partner. In that case, try to address the addiction before packing your bags and calling it quits.

Have "the talk" described at the beginning of this chapter. When discussing what your partner's goals are in life, include your joint goals as a loving team. Remind your partner of what the two of you used to dream of having together. And remind your partner that crystal is ruining not just his or her life, but also the life that the two of you have built together.

Protect Yourself

While you are trying to be compassionate and caring toward your partner, always be sure to take care of yourself. This is not being selfish. If you are not healthy or safe, you cannot help your partner. And if you are finding that your relationship is destructive to you, then in the long run it is hurtful to your partner, as well. Some things to keep in mind:

- If there is ever any violence or abuse, leave immediately.
- If your partner is using up all of your joint savings, then divide the money fairly into separate bank accounts and get rid of any joint credit cards. If you are financially dependent on him or her, you need to find a way to protect yourself financially or you may find yourself homeless because of your partner's addiction.
- If your partner is having sex outside the relationship, *always* use condoms when the two of you have sex.
- Get checked regularly by your doctor for sexually transmitted diseases.
- Get emotional support from friends, family, support groups, a therapist, or Al-Anon.

Set limits for yourself and your partner. What are you able to tolerate? What limits are healthy for the relationship? What limits do you need to address the crystal addiction? When you draw the line, be compassionate but firm. If necessary, seek the assistance of a couples' therapist who specializes in addiction.

In the end, the relationship may not survive, at least not in its present state, while your partner is heavily addicted. Losing a partner to crystal is painful, but hitting that rock bottom may eventually motivate that person to change and get help.

On the other hand, your relationship may survive. It will be different, and it may become even stronger than before as the two of you learn how to navigate the treacherous seas together. This requires communicating well, learning new ways to support each other, and understanding each other's needs more clearly. These are all assets that make any relationship stronger and deeper.

APPENDIX 1
Abstinence-Based Treatment and General Information Resources

THE FOLLOWING RESOURCES are facilities and Web sites that provide information and/or treatment for crystal addiction based on an abstinence-based model. Except for the twelve-step organizations, this list comprises programs that specifically have experience in working with methamphetamine addiction. There are many other excellent programs that offer general addiction treatment. This list does not guarantee the quality of the treatment of each facility or the accuracy of information presented in the Web sites. Therefore, use your own discretion and judgment when investigating these resources. When possible, some information is provided describing details of what these programs offer.

NATIONAL:

Al-Anon/Alateen
Provides information and locations of Al-Anon and Alateen meetings in the United States, Canada, and Puerto Rico.

Al-Anon Family Group Headquarters, Inc.
1600 Corporate Landing Parkway
Virginia Beach, VA 23454-5617
Phone: (757) 563-1600 Fax: (757) 563-1655

Al-Anon Family Group Headquarters, Inc.
(Canada)
9 Antares Drive, Suite 245
Ottawa, ON K2E 7V5
Phone: (613) 723-8484 Fax: (613) 723-0151

Al-Anon General Outreach
(888) 4AL-ANON or (888) 425-2666

Alateen (Al-Anon meetings specifically for teens with an addicted family member)
www.al-anon.alateen.org/meetings/meeting.html

Alcoholics Anonymous
AA World Services, Inc.
P.O. Box 459
New York, NY 10163
(212) 870-3400
www.alcoholics-anonymous.org

Crystal Meth Anonymous (CMA)
CMA General Services Chair
8205 Santa Monica Boulevard PMB 1-114
West Hollywood, CA 90046-5977
(213) 488-4455 (Hotline)
www.crystalmeth.org

A Key to Methamphetamine-Related Literature (Web site information resource)
An exhaustive, frequently updated list of literature on various aspects of methamphetamine published by the New York State Department of Health, AIDS Institute.
www.nyhealth.gov/diseases/aids/harm_reduction/crystalmeth/docs/meth_literature_index.pdf

KnowCrystal.org
Provides general information about crystal in a nonjudgmental way. This site does not offer treatment services.
www.KnowCrystal.org

National Institute of Drug Abuse
Neuroscience Center Building
6001 Executive Boulevard
Rockville, MD 20852
www.nida.nih.gov

United States Health and Human Services, Substance Abuse and Mental Health Service Administration (SAMHSA)
1 Choke Cherry Road
Rockville, MD 20850
Center for Substance Abuse Prevention (CSAP) (240) 276-2420
Center for Substance Abuse Treatment (CSAT) (240) 276-1660
www.samhsa.gov/index.aspx

CALIFORNIA:
AIDS Project LA (APLA) Crystal Methamphetamine Program
The David Geffen Center
611 South Kingsley Drive
Los Angeles, CA 90005
(213) 201-1600
www.apla.org/prevention/crystal_meth.html

Crystal Meth Treatment (Laguna Beach)
Treatment program for both gay and straight people with crystal-specific treatment
(800) 930-METH
www.crystalmethtreatment.com

Friends La Brea
Los Angeles
1134 N La Brea Avenue
West Hollywood, CA 90038
(323) 463-7001

S.T.O.P. (Stimulant Treatment Outpatient
    Program)
3180 18th Street, Suite 202
San Francisco, CA   94102
(415) 502-5777

San Francisco Lesbian/Gay/Bisexual/Trans-
    gender Community Center
1800 Market Street
San Francisco, CA 94102
(415) 865-5555

Van Ness Recovery House
Los Angeles
(323) 463-4266

FLORIDA:
Gay and Lesbian Community Center of
    South Florida
1717 N Andrews Avenue
Ft. Lauderdale, FL 33311
Phone (954) 463-9005   Fax (954) 764-6522
www.glccsf.org

MASSACHUSETTS:
Fenway Community Health Center
7 Haviland Street
Boston, MA 02115
(888) 242-0900

NEW YORK:
Callen-Lorde Community Health Center
326 West 18th Street
New York, NY 10011
(212) 271-7200
www.callen-lorde.org

Columbia University Medical Center Depart-
    ment of Psychiatry
(Frequently conducts studies that offer free
    treatment, including medication and
    therapy, for methamphetamine users with
    HIV. At the time this book is going to press,
    Columbia has a study offering treatment
    of methamphetamine addiction with
    modafinil combined with therapy.)
1051 Riverside Drive
New York, NY 10032
Contact persons: Dr. Judith Rabkin (212)
    543-5762 and Dr. Martin McElhiney (212)
    543-5331

The Crystal Clear Program at the Addiction
    Institute of New York (formerly known as
    the Smithers Treatment Institute)
1111 Amsterdam Avenue
New York, NY 10025
 (212) 523-6491

Gay Men's Health Crisis (GMHC)
120 W 20th Street
New York, NY 10011
General: (212) 807-6655
Hotline: (800) 243-7692
Substance Use Counseling and Education
information line: (212) 367-1354
www.gmhc.org/programs/suce.html

The Lesbian, Gay, Bisexual & Transgender
    Community Center
208 West 13th Street
New York, NY 10011
Phone: (212) 620-7310
Fax: (212) 924-2657
www.gaycenter.org

WASHINGTON, D.C.:
Whitman-Walker Clinic
1407 S Street, NW
Washington, DC 20009
(202) 797-3500
http://wwc.org/

APPENDIX 2
Harm-Reduction Resources

THE FOLLOWING RESOURCES are facilities and Web sites that provide information and/or treatment for crystal addiction based on a harm-reduction approach. Some of the facilities are also listed in Appendix 1 (abstinence-based treatment) because they offer both models of care. This list does not guarantee the quality of the treatment of each facility or the accuracy of the information provided by the individual Web sites. Use your own discretion and judgment when investigating these resources.

ATLANTA:
Atlanta Harm Reduction Center
(404) 526-9222
www.atlantaharmreduction.org

BOSTON:
Fenway Community Health Center
(617) 267-0900
www.fenwayhealth.org

CHICAGO:
The Chicago Recovery Alliance
www.anypositivechange.org

LOS ANGELES:
AIDS Project Los Angeles (APLA)
(213) 201.1600
www.apla.org

NEW YORK:
The Lesbian, Gay, Bisexual & Transgender
    Community Center
212-620-7310
www.gaycenter.org

Gay Men's Health Crisis (GMHC)
General Hotline: (800) 243-7692
    Substance Use Counseling and Education (S.U.C.E.) information line:
    (212) 367-1354
www.gmhc.org/programs/suce.html

Positive Health Project
301 West 37th Street, 2nd Floor
New York, NY 10018
(212) 465-8304, x33
tevans
Exclusive drop-in hours for gay and bisexual
    men with concerns about crystal
Fridays 5:00–8:00 p.m.

SALT LAKE CITY:
Harm Reduction Project
(801) 355-0234
www.harmredux.org

SAN FRANCISCO:
The Stonewall Project
 (415) 502-1999

Haight-Ashbury Free Clinics
(415) 565-1908
www.hafci.org

S.T.O.P. (Stimulant Treatment Outpatient
    Program)
 (415) 502-5777

San Francisco Lesbian/Gay/Bisexual/Trans-
    gender Community Center
(415) 865-5555
www.glccsf.org

WASHINGTON, D.C.:
Whitman-Walker Clinic
(202) 797-3500
http://wwc.org

GENERAL INFORMATION WEB SITES

www.tweaker.org
www.harmreduction.org
www.dancesafe.org
www.clubdrugcounselor.com
www.canadianharmreduction.com

GLOSSARY

abstinence: Completely stopping the use of a substance. This is in contrast to "moderation management," which is a philosophy that drug or alcohol use can be continued in a controlled and moderate way.

acamprosate: A medication that is used for alcoholism, thought to decrease the urge to drink by enhancing GABA transmission and decreasing overactive gluatamate activity at NMDA receptors. A recent large-scale study questioned whether acamprosate has actual benefit for alcoholics, finding its effect similar to a placebo. It is under investigation for use in other chemical addictions.

acute: Sudden onset. E.g., "acute pain" occurs suddenly, as opposed to "chronic pain," which is long lasting. An acute event, which starts suddenly, can become chronic if it continues for a long time

ADD: See attention-deficit/hyperactivity disorder

ADHD: See attention-deficit/hyperactivity disorder

amygdala: A part of the brain where emotional memory is stored.

anabolic steroids: A class of drugs that mimic testosterone and are used to treat hormone deficiencies, low libido, severe weight loss from HIV and cancer, and anemia. They are also misused by health people to promote muscle growth.

astrocyte: A type of cell in the brain that supports other brain cells that are responsible for thinking, feeling, and other basic "brain functions," by protecting, nourishing, and assisting their function

attention deficit disorder: See attention-deficit/hyperactivity disorder

attention-deficit/hyperactivity disorder: A psychiatric illness in which a person has difficulty with a number of mental functions, most notably focusing attention on uninteresting material and having difficulty filtering out surrounding distractions, having difficulty suppressing movements or words and needing to move about constantly. There are three subtypes: 1) primarily inattentive; 2) primarily hyperactive; and 3) combined inattentive and hyperactive. In adults, it is more common to see the primarily inattentive subtype, also commonly known as attention deficit disorder or ADD. Children are more commonly seen with the combined type. This condition is usually called by its simpler acronym ADHD. Note that there are many other conditions that can cause difficulty with concentration, such as depression, anxiety, drug effects, medication side effects, fatigue, and many others.

basal ganglia: A part of the brain with many functions, including movement, as well as relaying brain signals between the body and the rest of the brain. Commonly known illnesses such as Parkinson's disease and Huntington's disease originate here. Cells in the basal ganglia use dopamine as their primary means of communicating with other parts of the brain and body.

behavioral therapy: A type of psychotherapy that works on the assumption that physical and emotional reactions occur when one thing or event is paired with another. For example, the pairing of a computer with the event of smoking crystal causes the body and mind to have a reaction when seeing a computer, which then reminds the mind and body of feelings associated with smoking crystal. Behavior therapy works to extinguish the reaction by repeatedly exposing a person to one of the two things without the other until the associated reaction stops. In this example, exposing a person to a computer until the feelings about smoking crystal disappear, allowing a person to work at a computer safely without having overwhelming cravings to use drugs.

benzodiazepines: A class of medications that target the GABA receptors in the brain to decrease anxiety and to promote sleep. Benzodiazepines are habit-forming, meaning that after taking benzodiazepines for several weeks, the body becomes accustomed to their effect, and after they are stopped, sleep and anxiety worsen. In some cases, withdrawal can be severe, including extremely uncomfortable physical symptoms and possibly seizure.

booty bumping: Nickname for a method of using crystal by dissolving it in a small amount of liquid and squirting it into the rectum. Booty bumping is often done to enhance the experience of anal sex.

bottom: Nickname for a person who is the receptive partner in anal sex. This role occurs commonly in gay sex when a crystal user is not able to achieve an erection because of crystal but still wants to have sexual intercourse.

brain-reward circuit: A pathway in the brain that is highly associated with pleasure, compulsive repetition of behavior, and addiction. The more a drug stimulates this circuit, the more addictive it tends to be. The brain-reward circuit uses dopamine to function.

bullet: Nickname for a small bullet-shaped device used to discreetly dose and use small, measured doses of powdered drugs, such as crystal, cocaine, and ketamine.

bump: Nickname for a small amount of crystal or other powdered drug (cocaine, special K, etc.) that is snorted. A bump can be snorted from the tip of a small object, such as a a key, or from a snorting device nicknamed a "bullet."

Campral: Brand name for acamprosate.

carbohydrates: A class of foods made of small to large chains of sugar. This includes table sugar, fructose from fruits, potatoes, pasta, and rice.

carbs: Nickname for carbohydrates.

CD4 cells: A type of immune cell, a subgroup of T lymphocytes, also known as T-cells, that is responsible for signaling other immune cells to attack foreign invaders, such as viruses and bacteria. CD4 cells are also the target of HIV, which disables the central organizer of the immune system. In this way, HIV cripples the entire immune system.

CD4 count: A measure of the number of CD4 cells in a sample of blood, which is used as a measure of the health status of the immune system in people with HIV.

CD8 Cells: A type of immune cell, a subgroup of T lymphocytes, also known as T-cells that attack foreign invaders such as bacteria, parasites, and viruses. They are called into action by signals from CD4 cells, which stimulate them to multiply and attack the foreign invaders.

cerebral cortex: The outer wrinkled surface of the brain, which is where most of logical thinking and judgment are performed.

chronic: A chronic illness is a condition that has persisted for several months to years. This is in contrast to an "acute illness," which occurs suddenly and is usually brief, though an illness with an acute onset can become chronic if it continues and becomes a long-standing illness.

cingulum: A specific part of the brain that has been associated with motivation and initiating behavior.

circuit parties: Large dance parties with thousands of gay men held in cities throughout the world, where gay men travel from long distances to celebrate. These parties started as ways for closeted gay men to escape their homophobic communities and join an accepting group where homosexuality was not condemned. The association with a party gave the feeling of celebrating their sexual orientation. Drug use became extremely prevalent at these parties, where many gay men used this venue to "escape" the painful reality of living in a homophobic society. The understanding that social dictums such as the "evil" of homosexuality were not necessarily correct likely allowed gay men to challenge mainstream prohibitions against many drugs.

clean: A term used by the addiction community meaning "not using drugs or alcohol." It is possible to be "clean" but not "sober." See sober.

club drugs: Drugs commonly used at raves and circuit parties, usually referring to Ecstasy, ketamine, methamphetamine, and GHB.

cognitive therapy: A type of psychotherapy that focuses on correcting incorrect thoughts that lead to unwanted emotions or behaviors.

coming out: The act of telling someone that you are gay or bisexual. This includes "coming out to yourself," meaning admitting to yourself that you are gay or bisexual. This term comes from the expression "coming out of the closet," meaning coming out of hiding about your sexuality.

compulsion: A strong urge to do an action that creates intense and possibly intolerable anxiety until the action is done. E.g., the compulsion to use a drug, even after several months of not using the drug.

counselor: The general term for a person who works with you to assist you in achieving a particular goal. A counselor can be from almost any discipline—drug counselors, social workers, psychologists, and psychiatrists. However, in certain states, people can call themselves "counselors" without any licensing or regulation of the quality of their work. Find out the background and training of any counselor you work with.

crash: The period after using a drug, which is usually unpleasant, like a "car crash."

creatinine phosphokinase: A substance that is in muscles, which is released when there is muscle damage. Creatinine phosphokinase is toxic to the kidneys, and in large amounts can cause kidney failure.

cybersex: The activity of deriving sexual pleasure while communicating with another person over the Internet. Usually this involves masturbation and use of the Internet to achieve an orgasm, but this is not always necessary to gratify the sexual needs. Cybersex has also begun to refer to any Internet activity, such as viewing pictures or videos to achieve orgasm.

delirium tremens: A specific medical condition that can occur from alcohol withdrawal that includes severe confusion, disorientation, agitation, and hallucinations. This is a serious medical condition that is potentially fatal.

destigmatize: To take away the negative feelings that society has closely associated with something. E.g., destigmatizing addiction is important to allow addicted people to stop feeling shame and to be more willing to admit their problem and seek treatment.

detoxification (Detoxing): The process of stopping a drug (including alcohol) and allowing the body to adjust to functioning without the drug in the body.

Diagnostic and Statistical Manual, Fourth Edition: A manual published by the American Psychiatric Association that describes specific criteria for psychiatric illnesses.

dopamine: A chemical used by cells in the body to send signals to other cells that cause changes in body function. E.g., dopamine affects signals directing heart function, mood, movement, pleasure, concentration, and motivation.

dopamine transporter: A protein in the cell wall of brain cells that transports dopamine from the space outside brain cells back into the brain cell, where it can be packaged into vesicles for use again. The dopamine transporter is blocked by both cocaine and methamphetamine, allowing dopamine to accumulate and causing the high of the drugs.

dope-sick: The feelings of withdrawal when stopping an opiate, such as heroin, Vicodin, or OxyContin.

DSM-IV: See "Diagnostic and Statistical Manual, Fourth Edition."

dysthymia: A low-level depressed mood that persists most days of the year for several years.

Ecstasy: See methylenedioxymethamphetamine.

electrolytes: Atomic particles such as sodium, potassium, and calcium that are important for the proper functioning of cells in the entire body. Imbalances in electrolytes can have a significant effect on brain, heart, and kidney function.

free radicals: Chemically reactive particles that cause derangement of cellular DNA, damage cell function, and destroy cells in the body. Free radicals have been implicated in causing cancer, brain damage from drugs, and aging.

frontal cortex: The front part of the brain's surface, which is involved in higher-level thinking, such as logic, judgment, and decision making

gamma hydroxybutyrate: A drug usually ingested as a liquid, which suppresses brain activity, causing lowering of inhibitions, euphoria, increase in libido, and sedation. Known commonly as GHB, it is extremely dangerous because the amount to cause unconsciousness is only slightly higher than the amount required to cause the high. In overdose, or when combined with other brain-supressing drugs, such as alcohol, benzodiazepines, ketamine, and opiates, it can be fatal.

GHB: See gamma hydroxybutyrate

glutamate: A small particle called a neuropeptide that is used to send signals between cells throughout the brain. Glutamate is especially known for its use in the cerebral cortex, where logical thinking and judgments are processed.

HAART: See highly active antiretroviral treatment.

hallucinations: Perception of something that is not actually there. There can be hallucinations of any of the senses: visual (sight), auditory (sounds and voices), tactile (feeling things on the skin, such as crawling bugs), olfactory (smells), and gustatory (taste). People may be aware or unaware of the fact that hallucinations are not actually there.

harm reduction: A philosophy of addiction treatment that identifies and works towards the goals of the addict, rather than forcing the addict to take on goals assigned by the clinician. Harm reduction emphasizes self-motivation, self-reliance, and self-empowerment. It relies on the assumption that people can make logical choices about what to do if they are given enough information and education. This model works best in the early stages of crystal use, before neurological changes occur that disrupt the ability to make logical decisions regarding drug use.

helper T-cells: A specific type of immune cell, also known as CD4 cells, that recognize a foreign invader (e.g., bacteria, viruses, and parasites), and sends signals to other immune cells to activate them to multiply and destroy the foreign invaders. Helper T-cells are also the primary targets for HIV, which therefore destroys the immune system's ability to fight infections.

highly active antiretroviral treatment (HAART): A regimen of three or more medications that must be taken simultaneously to fight HIV, sometime referred to as an "HIV cocktail."

hypothalamus: A small area of the brain that secretes hormones, regulates body functions such as eating and sex, and controls the "body clock," telling your body when to sleep and awaken.

immune system: The system of cells and chemicals secreted by these cells that kill foreign invaders, such as bacteria, viruses, and parasites.

in vitro: A type of biological study that uses chemicals and/or cells but does not involve animals or humans. These studies are helpful, but animal studies are considered a better approximation of what happens in humans. Human studies are the best at showing what actually happens in people.

in vivo: A type of biological study that uses humans or other animals. These studies are considered a better reflection of activity in the human body, with human studies being the most accurate.

inpatient rehabilitation: Intensive drug addiction treatment in a hospital setting.

insight: Clear knowledge about oneself, one's thoughts, and one's behavior. E.g., a person can have good insight into the fact that he is addicted to crystal. Conversely, a person can have poor insight into his addiction and justify his weekly use as recreational and "totally under my control," though he has not been able to pass a weekend without crystal in six months.

ketamine: A "club drug" that is usually in crystalline white powder form, derived from a liquid drug used for injection. Ketamine is a drug used as a general anesthesia for surgery on children and on animals in veterinary medicine. Also called Special-K.

killer T-cells: A specific type of immune cell, also known as CD8 cells, that are activated by helper T-cells (CD4 cells) to multiply and destroy foreign invaders, such as bacteria, viruses, and parasites.

limbic system: A grouping of brain circuits that are linked and regulate emotions.

line: A rough measure of a powdered drug that is snorted. The powder is laid on a flat smooth surface and divided into lines of various lengths and widths. This is a very inexact measure because the size of the line can vary with the user, and as an addiction worsens, the size of one line can become much larger than it had been in previous years. Therefore the statement that "I do the same number of lines in a night as I used to" does not necessarily mean that drug use has not increased.

lymphocyte: A type of blood cell that is part of the immune system, which destroys foreign invaders, such as bacteria, viruses, and parasites.

major depression: See major depressive disorder.

major depressive disorder: A psychiatric illness in which a person has low mood, together with disturbed sleep, change in appetite, decreased energy and motivation, poor concentration, or a decreased ability to experience pleasure. A combination of some of these symptoms must be present for at least two weeks. This condition often responds well to treatment with antidepressant medication and psychotherapy. It can be worsened by crystal use and is also a condition that, when untreated, causes relapse to drug use.

Matrix Model: A model of treatment specifically tailored for people addicted to crystal.

MDMA: See methylenedioxymethamphetamine.

mesolimbic pathway: A brain pathway leading from the ventral tegmentum in the brainstem to the nucleus accumbuns in the brain. The mesolimbic pathway is associated with pleasure, as well as compulsive repetition of behaviors that may not necessarily be pleasurable.

meth mouth: A dental condition of softened, severely decayed teeth that results from poor nutrition and osteoporosis with weakened tooth structure; dry mouth, which increases bacterial growth that destroys teeth; and tooth grinding and jaw clenching caused by crystal

methylenedioxymethamphetamine (MDMA, or Ecstasy): Club drug that works on serotonin, taken in pill form. Ecstasy usually causes people to feel relaxed and takes away social anxieties and inhibitions.

modafinil: A medication used primarily to promote wakefulness with very little addiction potential. Modafinil has many actions, including increasing glutamate activity in the prefrontal cortex. It has been found to be helpful for cocaine addiction and is being investigated as a possible treatment for meth addiction. (Brand name Provigil.)

mu-opioid receptor: A subtype of receptor for opiates on cells in the brain and throughout the body. This subtype is most commonly known for its euphoric and pain-killing effects when opiates, such as heroin and morphine, are taken.

mushin: A Zen Buddhist concept meaning "no mind." Through mushin one tries to achieve a higher spiritual state by emptying the mind, which involves letting go of worries of the past and the future.

mutations and resistance: Changes that happen to the DNA (genes) in a virus or bacteria that make it resistant to medications that are used to effectively kill the virus or bacteria.

naltrexone: A medication that blocks opiate receptors, opposing the effect of opiates, such as heroin and morphine. It has been helpful in treating certain addictions, such as alcoholism and opiate dependence.

neocortex: The cerebral cortex, or outer covering of the brain in humans, which is a new (neo) evolutionary change that is present in human brains, when compared to the more primitive brains of other animals.

neurophysiologic: Pertaining to biological changes in nerve cells, particularly in the brain.

neurotransmitter: Chemicals used by brain cells and other nerve cells throughout the body to communicate with other nerve cells or parts of the body.

NMDA receptor: See N-methyl-D-aspartic acid receptor.

N-methyl-D-aspartic acid receptor: A protein in the cell wall of brain cells that is activated by glutamate to cause a series of subsequent actions within the brain cell. It is thought to be an important receptor in addiction, affecting cravings and the ability to make judgments necessary to avoid relapse.

nonoxynol-9: A chemical developed as a spermicide that is used in lubricants with condoms. Nonoxynol-9 had been found to kill HIV in test tubes, so it was recommended to use in lubricants to prevent HIV transmission. However, it was found to cause so much irritation to mucous membranes inside the rectum and vagina that it was thought to possibly make HIV transmission easier, so it is recommended that people not use lubricants containing nonoxynol-9.

norepinephrine: A neurotransmitter that has a stimulating effect. It is also called noradrenaline, which is more commonly known as adrenaline.

nucleus accumbens: An area in the brain that is associated with reward and addiction.

paranoia: A mental state in which a person falsely believes that others are following, watching, or in some way want to harm him.

Parkinson's disease: A neurological disorder affecting movement. The most prominent and common symptoms are tremor (shaking), expressionless face, and difficulty initiating a movement, such as walking or standing up from a chair. It is caused by damage to dopamine neurons in a part of the brain called the basal ganglia.

party (v. to party): A slang term meaning to use drugs, most often referring to using crystal.

PET scan: A test similar to X-rays and CAT scans that makes images of parts of the body. PET scans of the brain show how active different areas are during different activities, such as resting, concentrating, performing specific mental tasks, etc. PET scans are often used to compare the brain function of a particular group compared to the general population. E.g., PET scans can compare the brain function of crystal users to non–crystal users.

physiological: Referring to the biological workings of the body.

placebo: An inactive pill or other sham treatment used in research with animals and people to compare the effect of an actual treatment to a fake treatment, to rule out nonmedication effects, such as the power of suggestion that taking a pill will make an illness better.

PNP: Slang abbreviation for "party and play," referring to having sex while using crystal.

Positron emission tomography scan: See PET scan.

prefrontal cortex: A specific part of the cerebral cortex that is located in front of the part of the brain that controls movement. The prefrontal cortex is believed to coordinate thoughts, goals, and behavior. People who have damage to this area of the brain have been observed to intellectually know "right from wrong" but in their behavior, they act upon a strong need for immediate gratification. Therefore, proper functioning of this area of the brain is crucial for being able to maintain sobriety. Even if an addict intellectually knows that crystal use will destroy his life, he needs proper functioning of the prefrontal cortex to resist the urge for immediate gratification to use crystal again.

program, the: A slang term in Alcoholics Anonymous that refers to the process of recovery, which involves ongoing effort. To stay sober in recovery, one must "work the program."

protease inhibitor: A class of medications used to treat HIV. This class of medications is very powerful at fighting HIV, but it also interacts with many other medications and drugs. The interaction could result in a dangerously high level of drug in the body, or certain drugs and medications could result in a low level of protease inhibitor, which would then allow HIV to grow and multiply.

Provigil: Brand name for modafinil.

psychodynamic psychotherapy: A type of psychotherapy based on the principle that much of a person's behavior is motivated and controlled by thoughts and feelings in the unconscious (i.e., thoughts and feelings that are outside a person's awareness).

psychosis: a fundamental derangement of the mind (as in schizophrenia) characterized by defective or lost contact with reality especially as evidenced by delusions, hallucinations, and disorganized speech and behavior.

rationalizing: Trying to make excuses for doing something that you know is wrong. E.g., "Brian rationalized that he could do a little crystal because it had been several months since he had used any drugs, and he was entertaining friends he hadn't seen in four years. He didn't want to spoil the fun and thought doing a couple of bumps wouldn't be a problem."

rave: A large gathering of teenagers and young adults, from hundreds to thousands, where people dance to techno music. Raves are a setting in which use of club drugs is a normal part of the culture.

recovery: A state of actively trying to remain sober and in control of an addiction. "Alison has been an alcoholic since she was seventeen, but she has been in recovery for the past five years."

relapse: Falling back into drug use after achieving a period of sobriety.

relapse prevention: A type of addiction treatment with the ultimate goal of complete abstinence, using various practical techniques to avoid or prevent relapse.

remit, remitting: To resolve or get better. Addiction and hypertension are remitting and relapsing illnesses because they both get better with treatment, but they can worsen at times, and this is expected as part of the course of the illnesses.

residential rehabilitation: Similar to inpatient rehabilitation, residential rehabilitation is addiction treatment in a live-in setting, though not in a hospital. The advantage of residential rehabilitation is that it removes addicts from the environment full of stressors and triggers that would increase an addict's chance of relapsing, and it allows the addict to intensively devote full time and attention to achieving and maintaining sobriety.

Revia: Brand name for naltrexone.

rhabdomyolysis: A medical condition in which muscles break down at a rapid rate. This is extremely dangerous because muscle breakdown products are toxic to the kidneys and can cause kidney failure if not caught and treated quickly.

rock bottom: A frightening low-point in an addict's life that helps him to realize that his drug use is a serious problem that needs to stop.

seizure: Abnormal electrical discharges in the brain that can result in loss of consciousness and contraction of all muscles, followed by shaking of all parts of the body.

selective serotonin-reuptake inhibitor: A type of medication that block the reuptake of serotonin, allowing serotonin to accumulate around cells in the brain. These medications are used to treat depression, anxiety, social anxiety disorder, panic disorder, obsessive-compulsive disorder, post-traumatic stress disorder, and many other conditions. It is a nonaddictive treatment for these illnesses.

serotonin: A neurotransmitter known to be important in maintaining mood, anxiety, and certain aspects of thinking and memory.

sexual orientation: Attraction to people of the same, opposite, or both genders. This includes heterosexual, homosexual, and bisexual. Sexual orientation is different from gender identity, which is the inner sense of being male, female, or "other."

sexuality: A general term encompassing various aspects of a person's identity that relate to sex, including sexual orientation, gender identity, preferred sexual activities, etc.

slam: Slang term for using a drug intravenously.

sober: Not using drugs or alcohol. Sometimes the word sober also implies actively working on fighting addiction. E.g., the expression "Clean but not sober" means a person is not currently using drugs but is not "working the program" or actively working on keeping addiction under control.

sobriety: See sober.

social anxiety disorder: A psychiatric illness in which a person has a disabling reaction of anxiety when exposed to other people, usually with fearful thoughts of being scrutininzed and humiliated.

social phobia: See social anxiety disorder.

Special K: See ketamine.

SSRI: See selective serotonin-reuptake inhibitor.

stimulants: A class of medications and drugs that increase energy, decrease the need for sleep, and usually suppress appetite. These substances act primarily on dopamine and norepinephrine.

striatum: A part of the brain in the basal ganglia that deals with reward-linked motivation, planning, and impulse control.

subcortical dementia: A type of brain damage occurring in deeper parts of the brain. Subcortical dementia can result from various conditions, including high blood pressure, multiple sclerosis, HIV, and chronic use of drugs such as crystal.

thalamus: Relays motor, sensory, and emotional signals to different parts of the brain

therapist: A person who works with people to help them sort out problems. Therapists can be of various disciplines, such as drug counselors, clinical social workers, psychologists, and psychiatrists. Within each discipline, there are different styles of therapy, including cognitive therapy, which is very "here-and-now"; psychodynamic, which focuses on the effects of early childhood experiences on adult life; hypnotherapy; etc. In many states, there is no strict regulation on what constitutes a therapist; therefore, the quality of care you may receive can vary. If you find a therapist with good experience who works in a style that fits you well, he or she can be extremely helpful, especially in helping to guide you out of the grip of addiction, because a therapist can point out things that you may know but do not allow yourself to see. For example, when you start to rationalize and begin to fall back into drug use.

top: A slang term among gay men, which means the "active" person in a sexual couple. In anal sex, the "top" penetrates the "bottom."

trick: A slang term among gay men, which means a person that you meet for sex only. Similar to a "quickie" or a "hookup." A trick is a casual sex acquaintance, in contrast to a person you meet for ongoing dating.

triggers: Anything that causes a person to start wanting a drug. The expression "people, places, and things" refers to triggers to be aware of to protect yourself from relapsing.

tweak: A slang word used as a verb meaning "to use crystal." The adjective "tweaked" means high on crystal, and a "tweaker" is a person who uses crystal.

twelve-step programs: A type of program based on the original Alcoholics Anonymous (AA) model, comprising of twelve "steps" to achieving and maintaining sobriety. These programs strive for complete abstinence, are peer-led, and strictly adhere to anonymity. Twelve-step programs use the terms "God" and "Higher Power," though there are many people in these programs who are not Christian or religious. Some examples of twelve-step programs are Alcoholics Anonymous (AA), Crystal Meth Anonymous (CMA), Cocaine Anonymous (CA), Marijuana Anonymous (MA), Narcotics Anonymous (NA), and Overeaters Anonymous (OA). This model of group treatment can be adapted to most addictive and compulsive behaviors.

vagus nerve: A nerve that runs from the upper chest, through the neck, and connects to various parts of the brain. Stimulation of this nerve can cause many changes in the brain, including changes in mood, motivation, and thinking.

ventral tegmentum: A small area in the brainstem that is connected by nerve fibers to the nucleus accumbens. These signals are mediated by dopamine and are often associated with pleasure.

viral Load: The amount of a virus that is measured in the blood. This term is most commonly used in reference to HIV because it is a barometer for how healthy a person with HIV is. A low or "undetectable" viral load usually signifies that HIV infection is under good control.

withdrawal: A physiological state in which the body needs more of a drug. A body goes into withdrawal when it becomes accustomed to the presence of a drug. When the drug is no longer present, the body feels sick. A crystal addict in withdrawal can feel tired, depressed, hungry, anxious, and even suicidal. Symptoms of withdrawal vary for each particular drug.

works: A slang term for needles and syringes used to inject drugs such as crystal, cocaine, and heroin into the bloodstream (intravenous drug use).

REFERENCES
AND BIBLIOGRAPHY

Alcoholics Anonymous. *Research Update*. Hazelden Foundation. December 2004.

Amphetamine Use Is Associated with Increased HIV Incidence Among Men Who Have Sex with Men in San Francisco. *AIDS*. 2055. 19(13):1423–24.

Arria, A. M.; Derauf, C. Lagasse, L. L.; Grant, P.; Shah, R.; Smith, L.; Haning, W.; Huestis, M.; Strauss, A.; Grotta, S.D.; Liu, J.; and Lester, B. Methampetamine and Other Substance Use During Pregnancy: Preliminary Estimates From the Infant Development, Environment and Lifestyle (ISDEAL) Study. *Maternal and Child Health Journal*. January 5, 2006, 1–10 [Epub ahead of printing]

Arria, A. M.; Derauf, C.; Lagasse, Ll.; Grant, P.; Shah, R.; Smith, L.; Haning, W.; Huestis, M.; Strauss, A.; Grotta, S. D.; Liu, J.; and Lester, B. Methamphetamine and Other Substance Use During Pregnancy: Preliminary Estimates From the Infant Development, Environment, and Lifestyle (IDEAL) Study. *Maternal Child Health Journal*. January 2006, 1–10. [Epub ahead of printing]

Bagby, D. High-risk Sex Not More Common When Meeting Online. *New York Blade*. www.nyblade.com. March 11, 2005, 11.

Berger, D. Minocycline Shown to Have Protection for the Brain Against HIV. *Positively Aware*. July/August 2005, 49–50.

Boddigger, D. Methamphetamine Use Linked to Rising HIV Transmission. www.thelancet.com. April 2005, 365:1217–1218.

Bowers, D. Don't Fool Yourself. *HIV Plus*. August 2005, 33.

Breaking Up With Tina. *Open Press*. New York, September 29, 2005.

Brecht, M. L.; Greenwell, L.; and Anglin, M. D. Substance Use Pathways to Methamphetamine Use Among Treated Users. *Addictive Behavior*. May 2, 2006. [Epub ahead of printing]

Brecht, M. L.; O'Brien, A.; von Mayrhauser, C..; and Anglin, M. D. Methamphetamine Use Behaviors and Gender Differences. *Addictive Behaviors*, 2004. 29 (1): 89–106.

Brodie, J. D.; Figueroa, E.; Laska, E. M; and Dewey, S. L. Safety and Efficacy of Gamma-vynil GABA (GVG) for the Treatment of Methamphetamine and/or Cocaine Addiction. *Synapse*. February 2005, 55(2): 122–25 .

Brummelte, S.; Grund, T.; Czok, A.; Teuchert-Noodt, G.; and Neddens, J. Long-term Effects of a Single Adult Methamphetamine Challenge: Minor Impact on Dopamine Fibre Density in Limbic Brain Areas of Gerbils. *Behavioral Brain Function*. March 2006, 28; 2:12

Cadet, J. L.; Jayanthi, S.; and Deng, X. Speed Kills: Cellular and Molecular Bases of Methamphetamine-induced Nerve Terminal Degeneration and Neuronal Apoptosis. *Journal of Pharmacological Science*. July 2003, 92(3): 178–195.

Callen-Lorde Community Health Center–Metamphetamine Treatment Program. Brief Summary of Evaluation Outcomes. *The New York Academy of Medicine, Division of Health Policy,* 2006.

Cass, W. A.; Harned, M. E.; Peters, L. E.; Nath, A.; and Maragos, W. F. HIV-1 Protein Tat Potentiation of Methamphetamine-induced Decreases in Evoked Overflow of Dopamine in the Striatum of the Rat. *Brain Research*. September 12, 2003, 984(1–2): 133–42.

Catanzarite, V. and Stein, D. A. Crystal and Pregnancy: Methamphetamine -associated Maternal Deaths. *Western Journal of Medicine*. May 1995, 162(5): 454–57.

Chang, L.; Ernst, T.; Speck, O.; and Grob, C. Additive Effects of HIV and Chronic Methamphetamine Use on Brain Metabolite Abnormalities. *Am Journal of Psychiatry*, 2005, 162: 361–369.

Chapa, S. War on Drugs Pushing Meth Labs South of the Border. *The Brownsville Herald*. www.brownsvilleherald.com/print.php?id=66571_0_10_0.

Chapman, D. E.; Hanson, G. R.; Kesner R. P.; and Keefe, K. A. Long-term Changes in Basal Ganglia Functioin After a Neurotoxic Regimen of Methamphetamine. *Journal of Psychopharmacological Experimental Therapies*, February 2001, 296(2): 520–27.

Cherner, M.; Letendre, S.; Heaton, R. K.; Durelle, J.; Marquie-Beck, J.; Gragg, B.; and Grant, A. Hepatits C Augments Cognitive Deficits Associated with HIV Infection and Methamphetamine. *Neurology*. April 7, 2005. [Epub ahead of printing]

Chicago Department of Public Health, STD/AIDS Chicago, Summer 2005.

Clemens, N. Desert Morning News.

Conant, K.; St. Hillaire, C.; Anderson, C.; Galey, D.; Wang, J.; and Nath, A. Human Immunodeficiency Virus Type 1 Tat and Metamphetamine Affect the Release and Activation of Matrix-degrading Proteinases. *Journal of Neurovirology*, February 2004, 10(1): 21–28.

Costello, D. Remix Cold Meds Pack Less Punch; Some Drug Companies Eliminate Ingredients That Are Used to Make Methamphetamines. *Los Angeles Times*. August 15, 2005. http://latimes.com/features/health/la-he-cold15aug15,1,7870165.story.

Cox. S. Risky Business. *Publication ACRIA Update*. Winter 2005/2006.

Curtis, P. Amphetamines Affect Men More Than Women. *Guardian*, April 8, 2006.

Czub, S.; Koutsilieri, E.; Sopeer, S.; Czub, M.; Stahl-Hennig, C.; Muller, J. G.; Pedersen, V.; Gesell, W.; Heeney, J. L.; Gerlach, M.; Gosztonyi, G.; Riederer, P.; Meulen, V. Enhancement of Central Nervous System Pathology in Early Simian Immunodeficiency Virus Infection by Dopaminergic Drugs. *Acta Neuropathology* (Berlin). February 2001, 101(2): 85–91.

D.C. Department of Health, Whitman-Walker Clinic Release Public Service Ad Aimed at Stemming Crystal Meth Use: 'Party'n'Pay' Targets Gay Men Using Chat Rooms, Bars. *Whitman-Walker Clinic Press Release*. March 14, 2006.

Davey, M. Grisly Effect of One Drug: 'Meth Mouth.' *New York Times*, June 11, 2005.

Denizet-Lewis, B. An Anti-Addiction Pill? *New York Times Magazine*. June 25, 2006. http://www.nytimes.com/2006/06/25/magazine/25addiction.html?ex=1152417600&en=5e28b4f74e295f51&ei=5070

Ellis, R. J Childers, M. E.; Cherner, M; Lazzaretto, D.; Letendre, S.; Grant, I.; and HIV Neurobehavioral Research Group. Increased Huma Immunodeficiency Virus Loads in Active Methamphetamine Users Are Explained by Reduced Efectiveness of Antiretroviral Therapy.

Journal of Infectious Diseases. December 15, 2003, 188(12): 1820–6.

Flora, G.; Lee, Y. W.; Nath, A.; Hennig, B.; Maragos, W.; and Toborek, M. Methamphetamine Potentiates HIV-1 Protein-mediated Activation of Redox-sensitive Pathways in Discrete Regions of the Brain. *Exp. Neurol.* January 2003, 179(1): 60–70.

Gavrilin, M. A.; Mathes, L. E.; and Podell, M. Methamphetamine Enhances Cell-associated Feline Immunodeficiency Virus Replication in Astrocytes. *Journal of Neurovirology*. June 2002, 8(3): 240–49.

Gibbie, T.; Mijch, A.; Ellen, S; Hoy, J.; Hutchison, C.; Wright, E.; Chua, P.; and Judd, F. Depression and Neurocognitive Performance in Individuals With HIV/AIDS: 2- year Follow-up. *HIV Medicine*. March 2006, 7(2):112–21.

Gordon, R. Study Confirms Role of Meth in HIV. *San Francisco Chronicle*, August 18, 2005.

Graham, C. Back on the Brink. *The Advocate*. September 27, 2005, 48–57.

Halkitis, P. N.; Green, K. A.; and Mourgues, P. Longitudinal Investigation of Methamphetamine Use Among Gay and Bisexual Men in New York City: Findings from Project BUMPS. *Journal of Urban Health*. March 2005, 82(1 Supl. 1): i18–25. Epub February 28, 2005.

Halkitis, P.N.; Parsons, J.T.; and Stirratt, M.J. A Double Epidemic: Crystal Methamphetamine Drug Use in Relation to HIV Transmission Among Gay Men. *Journal of Homosexuality*, 2001; 41(2): 17–35

Halkitis, P. N.; Shrem, M. T. Psychological Differences Between Binge and Chronic Methamphetamine Using Gay and Bisexual Men. *Addictive Behavior*, June 17, 2005. [Epub ahead of printing]

Hananel, S. Lawmakers Tangle Over Anti-Meth Legislation. *Associated Press*. September 27, 2005.

Henry J. Kaiser Family Foundation. HIV Infection May Cause Neurological Damage Regardless of Antiretroviral Therapy Effectiveness, Study Says. *The Body PRO, Medical News,* November 18, 2003.

Henry J Kaiser Family Foundation. Meth Use, HIV Infection Linked to Changes in Brain Structure That Can Impair Cognitive Functions, Study Says. *The Body PRO*, Newsroom, August 15, 2005.

HHS Awards $16.2 Million for Methamphetamine Abuse Treatment. *SAMHSA Advisory*. August 18, 2005.

Holtzman, D. Possible Link Found Between Cocaine and Susceptibility to PD. *CNS News*. March 2006, 35.

Huber, A.; Lord, R. H.; Gulati, V.; Marinelli-Casey, P.; Rawson, R.; and Ling, W. The CSAT Methamphetamine Treatment Program: Research Design Accommodations for 'Real World' Application. *Journal of Psychoactive Drugs*, April–June 2000, 32(2): 149–56.

Hythiam, Inc. Hythiam's PROMETA™ Protocols Featured in Article on Addiction in The New York Times Magazine on Sunday, June 24th. *Press Release*. June 26, 2006.

Illinois: Howard Brown Health Center Starts Crystal Meth Program. *CDC HIV, STD, TB Prevention News Update*. Http://www.the-body.com/cdc/news_pudates_archive/2005/nov18_05/ November 18, 2005.

IOWA Limits on Cold Medicines Lead to Major Drop in Meth Labs. Http://jointogether.org/y/0,2521,577831,00.html.

Jeng, W.; Ramkissoon, A.; Parman, T.; and Wells, P.G. Prostaglandin H Synthase-catalyzed Bioactivation of Amphetamines to Free Radical Intermediates That Cause CNS Regional DNA Oxidation and Nerve Terminal Degeneration. *FASB Journal*, April 2006, 20(6): 638–50

Jernigan, T. L.; Gamst, A. C.; Archibald, S. L.; Fennema-Notestine, C.; Rivera Mindt, M.; Marcotte, T.L.; Heaton, R.K.; Ellis, R.j.; and Grant, I. Effects of Methamphetamine Dependence and HIV Infection on Cerebral Morphology. *American Journal of Psychiatry*, August 2005, 162: 1461–72.

Kalivas, P. W.; and Volkow, N. D. Addiction Biology Suggests How to Block Relapse. *American Journal of Psychiatry*, August 2005, 162: A38.

Kalivas, P. W.; and Volkow, N. D. Do Brain Effects of HIV and Meth Cancel Each Other Out? *American Journal of Psychiatry*, August 2005, 162: A38.

Kalivas, P. W.; and Volkow, N. D. The Neural Basis of Addiction: A Pathology of Motivation and Choice. *American Journal of Psychiatry*, August 2005, 162: 1403–13

Kingston, S.; and Drug Use and HIV Prevention Team, Public Health-Seattle and King County. When Your Partner Has a Drug or Alcohol Problem: A Guide for Gay and Bisexual Men. September 2005.

Kita, T.; Wagner, G. C.; and Nakashime, T. Current Research on Methamphetamine-induced Neurotoxicity: Animal Models of Monoamine Disruption. June 2002, 965: 225–32.

Klasser, G. D.; Epstein, J. Methamphetamine and Its Impact on Dental

Care. *Journal of the Canadian Dental Association*. November 2005, 71(10): 756–62.

Knowing Reiki. http://www.salondereiki.com. Accessed August 20, 2005.

Krawczyk, C. S.; et al. Methamphetamine Use and HIV Risk Behaviors Among Heterosexual Men—-Preliminary Results from Five Northern California Counties. *Morbidity and Mortality Weekly Report*. March 17, 2006.

Kurtz, S. P. Post-circuit Blues: Motivations and Consequences of Crystal Meth Use Among Gay Men in Miami. *AIDS Behavior*. March 2005, 9(1): 63–72.

Lampinen, T.; McGhee, D.; and Martin, I. Use of Crystal Methamphetamine and Other Club Drugs Among High School Students in Vancouver and Victoria. *BC Medical Journal*, January/ February 2006, 48:1: 22–27.

Lampinen, T. M.; McGhee, D.; and Martin, I. Increased Risk of 'Club' Drug Use among Gay and Bisexual High School Students in British Columbia. *Journal of Adolescent Health*, April 2006, 38(4): 458–61.

Langford D.; Adame, A; Grigorian A.; Grant, I.; McCutchan, J. A.; Ellis, R. J.; Marcotte, T. D.; Masliah E.; and HIV Neurobehavioral Research Center Group. Patterns of Selective Neuronal Damage in Methamphetamine-user AIDS Patients. *Journal of Aquired Immune Deficiency Syndrome*. December 15, 2003, 34(5): 467–74.

Langford, D.; Grigorian, A.; Hurford, R.; Adame, A.; Crews, L.; and Masliah, E. The Role of Mitochondrial Alterations in the Combined Toxic Effects of Human Immunodeficiency Virus Tat Protein and Methamphetamine on Calbindin Positive-neurons. *Journal of Neurovirology*. December 2001, 10(6): 327–37.

Larimer, M. E.; Palmer, R. S.; and Marlatt, G. A. Relapse Prevention: An Overview of Marlatt's Cognitive-behavioral Model. *Alcohol Research and Health*, No 2, 1999, 23:151–60.

Lee, S. J.; Galanter, M.; Dermatis, H.; and McDowell, D. Circuit Parties and Patterns of Drug Use in a Subset of Gay Men. *Journal of Addictive Diseases*, 2003; 22(4): 47–60.

Levounis, P; and Ruggiero, J. S. Outpatient Management of Crystal Methamphetamine Dependence Among Gay and Bisexual men: How Can It Be Done? *Primary Psychiatry*. February 2006, 13(2): 75–80.

Lile, J. A.; Stoops, W. W.; Vansickel, A. R.; Glaser, P. E.; Hays, L. R.; and Rush, C. R. Ariprazole Attenuates the Discriminative-stimulus and Subject-rated Effects of D-amphetamine in Humans. *Neuropsychopharmacology*. November 2005, 30(11): 2103–14.

Lloyd, J. Methamphetamine. *Office on National Drug Control Policy, Drug Policy Information Clearinghouse*. Fact Sheet. November 2003, 1–6.

Long-term Methamphetamine Abuse Impairs Selective Inhibition. *NewsScan, NIDDA Addiction Research News*. August 23, 2005.

Maragos, W. F.; Young, K. L.; Turchan, J. T; Guseva, M.; Pauly, J. R.; Math, A.; and Cass, W. A. Human Immunodeficiency Virus-1 Tat Protein and Methamphetamine Interact Synergistically to Impair Striatal Dopaminergic Function. *Journal of Neurochmeistry*. 2002 November, 83(4): 955–63.

McGregor, C.; Srisurapanont, M.; Jittiwutikarn, J.; Laobhripatr, S.; Wongtan, T.; and White, J. M. The Nature, Time Course and Severity of Methamphetamine Withdrawal. *Addiction*. March 16, 2005, 100: 1320–29.

Meth is HIV Hazard Among Straight Men—Study Finds Users in Low-Income Areas Engage in Risky Sex. *HRP News Digest*. March 20, 2006.

Meth Use is Boosting HIV Rates in Denver. *Advocate.com*. March 16, 2006. http://www.advocate.com/print_article_ektid28034.asp

Methamphetamine Straining ED's, Treatment System. *ASAM News*. January–February 2006, 21: 1–3.

Methamphetamine. Executive Office of the President. Office of National Drug Control Policy. November 2003.

Nath, A.; Anderson, C.; Jones, M.; Maragos, W.; Booze, R.; Mactutus, C.; Bell, J.; Hauser K. F.; and Mattson, M. Neurotoxicity and Dysfunction of Dopaminergic Systems Associated with AIDS Dementia. *Journal of Psychopharmacology*. 2000, 14(3): 222–27.

Nath, A.; Hauser, KF.. Wojna, V.; Booze, R. M; Maragos, W.; Prendergast, M; Cass, W.; and Turchan, J. T. Molecular Basis for Interactions of HIV and Drugs of Abuse. *Journal of Acquired Deficiency Syndrome*. October 1, 2002. Suppl 2: S62–9.

New York Medical College; HIV-AIDS Education and Training, St. Vincent's Hospital Comprehensive HIV Center; Weill-Urbina, A.

(1–2); and Jones, K. (3–4). Crystal Methamphetamine, Its Analogues, and HIV Infection: Medical and Psychiatric Aspects of an Epidemic. Cornell Medical College; and Center for Special Studies, New York-Presbyterian Hospital, New York City. *Clinical Infectious Diseases*, 2004, 38: 890–94.

Newton, T. F.; Roache, J. D.; De La Garza, R. 2nd; Fong, T.; Wallace, C. L.; Li, S. H.; Elkashef, A.; Chiang, N.; and Kahn, R. Safety of Intravenous Methamphetamine Administration During Treatment with Bupropion. *Psychopharmacology (Berlin)*. November 2005, 182(3): 426–35. Epub October 19, 2005.

NIDA Unveils Campaign to Send Teens the Message About the Link Between Drug Abuse. And HIV. *NIH News*. November 29, 2005. http://www.nih.gov/news/pr/nov2005/nida-29.htm (accessed November 30, 2005)

O'Connor, Anahad. Scientists Explore Meth's Role in Immune System. New York Times. *The Body: The Complete HIV/Aids Resource*. February 25, 2005.

Office of National Drug Control Policy. Bush Cabinet Officials Highlight Administration Anti-Meth Programs. www.MethResources.gov.

Ornstein, C. Meth Users Respond to Reward Program. *Los Angeles Times*. http://archives.seattletimes.nwsource.com/cgi-bin/texis.cgi/web/vortex/display?slug=meth28&date=20051228&query=meth.

Ornstein, C. Meth Use by HIV-positive Men Rising: LA Clinic Study Shows Almost a Third of Gay and Bisexual Men Found to Have the Aids-causing Virus Last Year Admitting Using the Drug. *Los Angeles Times*. June 16, 2005. http://www.latines.com/news/local/la-me-aids16jun16,1,2276436.story.

Osborne, D. Forum Men Walk the Walk: Rising Infection Rates Impel Activists to Pay for Ads and Speak Out. *Gay City News*. November 27–December 3, 2003. 2:47. http://www.gaycitynews.com/gcn_248/forummenwalk.html.

Patterson, T. L.; and Semple, S. J. Sexual Risk Reduction Among HIV-positive Drug-using Men Who Have Sex With Men. *Journal of Urban Health*. December 2003, 80(4 Suppl 3): iii77–87.

Peck, J. A.; Reback, C. J.; Yang, X.; Rotheram-Fuller, E.; and Shoptaw, S. Sustained Reductions in Drug Use and Depression Simptoms from Treatment for Drug Abuse in Methamphetamine-dependent Gay and

Bisexual Men. *Journal of Urban Health*. March 2005. (1 Suppl 1): i100–i108. Epub 2005 Feb 28.

Peirce, J.; Petry, N.; Stitzer, M.; Blaine, J.; Kellogg, S.; Satterfield, F.; Schwartz, M.; Krasnansky, J.; Pencer, E.; Silva-Vazquez, L.; Kirby, K.; Royer-Malvestuto, C.; Roll, J.; Cohen, A.; Copersoine, M.; Kolodner, K.; and Li, R. Effects of Lower-Cost Incentives on Stimulant Abstinence in Methadone Maintenance System. *Arch Gen Psychiatry*. February 2006. 63: 201-208.

Petry, N.; Peirce, N.; Slitzer, M.; Blaine, J.; Roll, J.; Cohen, A.; Obert, J.; Kileen, T.; Saladin, M.; Cowel, M.; Kirby, K.; Sterling. R.; Royer-Malvestuto, C.; Hamilton, J.; Booth, R.; MacDonald, M.; Liebert, M.; Rader, L.; Burns, R.; DiMaria, J.; Copersino, M.; Quinn Stabile, P.; Kolodner, K.; and Li, R. Effect of Prize-Based Incentives on Outcomes in Stimulant Abusers in Outpatient Psychosocial Treatment Programs. *Arch Gen Psychiatry*. October 2005, 62: 1148–56. www.archgenpsychiatry.com.

Phillips, T. R.; Billaud, J. N.; and Henriksen, S. J. Methamphetamine and HIV-1: Potential Interactions and the Use of the FIV/Cat Model. *Journal of Psychopharmacology*, 2000, 14(3): 244–50.

Rabkin, J. G.; McElhiney, M. C.; Rabkin, R.; and Ferrando S. J. Modafinil Treament for Fatigue on HIV+ Patients: A Pilot Study. *Journal of Clinical Psychiatry*. December 2004, 64(12): 1688–95.

Ramamoorthy, J. D.; Ramamoorthy, S.; Leibach, F. H.; and Ganapathy, V. Human Placental Monoamine Transporters as Targets for Amphetamines. *American Journal of Obstetrics and Gynecology*. December 1995, 173(6): 1782–87.

Rawson, R. A.; Gonzalez, R.; Obert, J. L.; McCann, M. J.; and Brethen, P. Methamphetamine Use Among Treatment-seeking Adolescents in Southern California: Participant Characteristics and Treatment Response. *Journal of Substance Abuse Treatment*. September 2005, 29(2): 67–74.

Reback, C. J; Larkins, S; and Shoptaw, S. Methamphetamine Abuse as a Barrier to HIV Medication Adherence Among Gay and Bisexual Men. *AIDS Care*. December 2003, 15(6): 775–85.

Recommendations from the CDC Consulation on Methamphetamine Use and Sexual Risk Behavior for HIV/ STD Transmission. Centers for Disease Control and Prevention. January 13–14, 2005, 1–9.

Reichard, J. Small Rewards Bring Sizable Payoff in Program to Keep Drug Abusers Off Cocaine, Methamphetamine. CQ *Healthbeats News*. October 13, 2005.

Research Across America. Study of PROMETA Protocol Shows Clinical Effectiveness: Statistically Significant Reduction in Methamphetamine Cravings and Methamphetamine Use. *Press Release*. June 21, 2006.

Reuters Health. Methamphetamine Use Curbs Efficacy of HAART For HIV Infection. *Journal of Infectious Diseases*, 2003, 188:1820–26.

Rippeth, J. D.; Heaton, R. K.; Carey, C. L.; Marcotte, T. D.; Moore, D. J.; Gonzalez, R.; Wolfson, T.; Grant, I.; and HNRC Group. Methamphetamine Dependence Increases Risk of Neuropsychological Impairment in HIV Infected Persons. *Journal of International Neuropsychology Society*. January 2004, 10(1): 1–14.

Scheller, C.; Sopper, S.; Jassoy, C.; Ter Meulen, V.; Riederer, P; and Koutsilieri, E. Dopamine Activates HIV in Chronically Infected T Lymphoblasts. *Journal of Neural Transmission*. 2000, 107(12): 1483–89.

Selnes, O. A. Memory Loss in Persons with HIV/AIDS: Assessment and Strategies for Coping. *AIDS Reading*, June 2005, 15(6): 293.

Sekine, Y.; Ouchi, Y.; Takei, N.; Yosikawa, E.; Nakamura, K.; Futatsubashi, M.; Okada, H.; Minabe, Y.; Suzuki, K.; Iwata, Y.; Tsuchiya, K.; Tsukada, H.; Iyo, M.; and Mori, N. Brain Serotonin Transporter Density and Aggression in Abstinent Methamphetamine Abusers. *Arch Gen Psychiatry*. 2006, 63:90–100.

Semple, D. J; Grant, I.; and Patterson, T. L. Female Methamphetamine Users: Social Characteristics and Sexual Risk Behavior. *Women's Health*. 2004, 40(3): 35–50.

Semple, D. J.; Zians, J.; Grant, I.; and Patterson. T. L. Impulsivity and Methamphetamine Use. *Journal of Substance Abuse Treatment*. September 2005, 29(2): 85–93.

Semple, S. J.; Grant, I; and Patterson T. L. Negative Self-Perceptions and Sexual Risk Behavior Among Heterosexual Methamphetamine Users. *Substance Use & Misuse*. 2005, 40(12): 1797–810.

Semple, S. J.; Patterson, T. L.; and Grant, I. The Context of Sexual Risk Behavior Among Heterosexual Methamphetamine Users. *Addictive Behavior*. June 2004, 29(4): 807–810.

Shoptaw, S.; Huber, A.; Peck, J.; Yang, X.; Liu, J.; Dang, J.; Roll, J.; Schapiro, B.; Rotheram-Fuller, E.; and Ling, W. Randomized, Placebo-controlled Trial of Sertraline and Contingency Mangement for the Treatment of Methamphetamine Dependence. *Drug and*

Alcohol Dependence. 2006. Article in press. www.elsevier.com/locate/drugalcdep.

Shoptaw, S.; Peck, J.; Reback, C.J.; Rotheram-Fuller, E. *Journal of Psychoative Drugs.* May 2003; 35 Suppl 1: 161–8.

Simao, P. Internet Fuels Risky Sex in Gay, Bisexual Men.*The Body.* June 16, 2005. http://www.thebdy.com/cdc/news_updates_archive/2005/jun16_05/.

Slamberova, R.; and Rokyta, R. Seizure Susceptibility in Prenatally Methamphetamine-exposed Adult Female Rats. *Brain Research.* October 26, 2005, 1060 (1–2): 193–7.

Slamberova, R.; Pometlova, M.; and Charousova, P. Postnatal Development of Rat Pups Is Altered By Prenatal Methmaphetamine Exposure. *Progress in Neuropsychopharmacological and Biological Psychiatry.* January 2006, 30(1); 82–8. Epub 2005 July 19.

Sommerfeld, J. Beating an Addiction to Meth: Researchers Zero In on Brain Effects, Treatment Approaches. *MSNBC.* http://www.msnbc.msn.com/id/3076519/print/1/displaymode/1098/.

State and Local Leaders Call for Action on Alarming New Latino HIV/AIDS Trends. *Bienestar* (Press Release, March 21, 2006.

Stewart, J. L. and Meeker, J. E Fetal and Infants Deaths Associated with Maternal Methamphetamine Abuse. *Journal of Analytical Toxicology.* October 1997, 21(6): 515–17.

Stoops, W. W.; Lile, J. A.; Glaser, P. E.; and Rush, C. R. A Low Dose of Ariprazole Attenuates the Subject-rated Effects of D-amphetamine. *Drug and Alcohol Dependence.* March 13, 2006. [Epub ahead of printing]

Taylor, M.; Aynalem, G.; Simth, L.; Bemis, C.; Keeney, K. and Kerndt P. Correlates of Internet Use to Meet Sex Partners Among Men Who Have Sex with Men Diagnosed with Early Syphilis in Los Angeles County. *Sexually Transmitted Diseases.* September 2004, 31:9: 552–56.

The 2004 National Survey on Drug Use and Health. *Substance Abuse and Mental Health Services Association* (SAMHSA), September 8, 2005. http://www.samsa.gov/news/newsreleases/050901_survey.htm.

The Matrix Model. National Institute on Drug Abuse. Behavioral Therapies Development Program-Effective Drug Abuse Treatment Approaches.

Treatment Admissions Increase for Methamphetamine and Narcotic Pain Medications in 2003. *SAMHSA E-news Release*, July 18, 2005.

Truong, J. G.; Wilkins, D. G.; Baudys, J.; Croucj, D. J.; Johnson-

Davis, K. L.; Gibb, J. W.; Hanson, G. R.; and Fleckenstein, A. E. Age-dependent Methamphetamine-induced Alterations in Vesicular Monoamine Transporter-2 Function: Implications for Neurotoxicity. *Journal of Phamacological Experimental Therapies*, September 2005, 314(3): 1087–92. Epub May 18, 2005.

Turner, A. Crystal Meth's Comeback a Lethal Dose for Gay Men. *Houston Chronicle*, June 21, 2005. http://www.chron.com/cs/CDA/ ssitory.mpl/front/3233892.

Two-thirds of Ice Users 'Hooked': Study, *Sidney Morning Herald*. October 26, 2005. http://www.smh.com.au/news/NATIONAL/Twothirds-of-ice-users-ho...

U.S National Institute on Drug Abuse. Methamphetamine Abuse, HIV Infection Cause Changes in Brain Structure. *The Body*, August 11, 2005, http://www.thebody.com/nida/meth_brain.html,

Urbina, A. and Jones, K. Crystal Methamphetamine, Its Analogues, and HIV Infection: Medical and Psychiatric Aspects of a New Epidemic. *Clinical Infectious Diseases*, March 15, 2004, 38(6): 890–94. Epub 2004 Mar 1.

Vance, D. E. and Burrage, J. W. Jr. Sleep Disturbances and Psychomotor Decline in HIV. *Perceptual and Motor Skills*. June 2005. 100(3 Pt 2):1004–10.

Vazquez, E. Crystal Meth Recovery: A Step-by-Step Guide. *Positively Aware*, September/ October 2005, 20–25.

Virmani, A.; Gaetani, M. F.; Imam, S.; Binienda, Z.; and Ali, S. The Protective Role of L-carnitine Against Neurotoxicity Evoked by Drug of Abuse, Methamphetamine, Could Be Related to Mitochondrial Dysfunction. *Annals of New York Academy of Science*, June 2002, 965: 225–32.

Virmani, A.; Gaetani, F.; Imam, S.; Binienda Z.; and Ali, S. The Proctective Role of L-Carnitine Against Neurotoxicity Evoked by Drug of Abuse, Methamphetamine, Could Be Related to Mitochondrial Dysfunction. *Journal of Pharmacology*, February 2001, 292(2): 520–27.

Vocci, F. and Ling, W. Medications Development: Success and Challenges. *Pharmacology and Therapeutics*, October 2005, 108(1): 94–108.

Vorhees, C. V.; Reed, T. M.; Morford, L. L.; Fukumura, M.; Wood, S. L.; Brown, C. A.; Skelton, M. R.; McCrea, A. E.; Rock, S. L.; and Williams, M. T. Periadolescent Rats (P41–50) Exhibit Increased

Susceptibility to D-Methamphetamine-induced Long-term Spatial and Sequential Learning Deficits Compared to Juvenil, (P21–30 or P31–40) or Adult Rats (P51–60). *Neurotoxicology and Teratology,* January-February 2005, 27(1): 117–34.

Wertheimer, A. L.; Cahney, N. M.; and Santella, T. Counterfeit Pharmaceuticals: Current Status and Future Projections. *Journal of American Pharmacology Association,* November-December 2003, 43(6): 710–7.

Whitten, L. Community-based Treatment Benefits Methamphetamine Abusers. *NIDA Notes,* 2006, 20(5): 4–5.

Whitten, L. Treatment Curbs Methamphetamine Abuse Among Gay and Bisexual Men. *NIDA Notes,* 20: 4:4–7.

Woody, G. E.; VanEtten-Lee, M. L.; McKirnan, D.; Donell, D.; Metzger, D.; Sea, G. 3rd; Gross, M.; and HIVNET 001 Protocol Team. Substance Use Among Men Who Have Sex with Men: Comparison with a National Household Survey. *Journal of Acquired Immune Deficency Syndrome,* May 1st, 2001, 27(1): 86–90.

Wu, L. T.; Schlenger, W. E.; and Galvin, D. M. Concurrent Use of Methamphetamine, MDMA, LSD, Ketamine, GHB, and Flunitrazepam among American Youths. *Drug and Alcohol Dependency,* February 14, 2006, [Epub ahead of printing]

Yen, C. F.; and Chong, M. Y. Comorbid Psychiatric Disorders, Sex, and Methamphetamine Use in Adolescents: a Case-Control Study. *Comprehensive Psychiatry,* May–June 2006, 47(3): 215–20.

Yen, C. F.; and Shieh, B. L. Suicidal Ideation and Correlates in Taiwanese Adolescent Methamphetamine Users. *Journal of Nervous Mental Disorders,* July 2005, 193(7): 444–49.

Yen, C. F.; and Su, Y. C. The Associations of Early-onset Methamphetamine Use with Psychiatric Morbidity among Taiwanese Adolescents. *Substance Use and Misuse,* 2006, 41(1): 35–44.

Yen, C. F.; Yang, Y. H.; Chong, M. Y. Correlates of Methamphetamine Use for Taiwanese Adolescents. *Psychiatry Clinical Neuroscience,* April 2006, 60(2): 160–67.

Young, E. Living With(out) Crystal Meth. *Positively Aware,* July/August 2005, 36–46.

Yu, Q.; Larson, D. F.; and Watson, R. R. Heart Disease, Methamphetamine and AIDS. *Life Science,* May 30, 2003, 73(2): 129–40.

Yu, Q.; Zhang, D.; Walston, M.; Zhang, J.; Liu, Y.; and Watson,

R. R. Chronic Methamphetamine Exposure Alters Immune Function in Normal and Retrovirus-infected Mice. *International Immunopharmacology*, June 2002, 2(7): 951–62.

Yu, Q.; Zhang, D.; Walston M.; Zhang, J.; Liu, Y.; and Watson, R. R. Chronic Methamphetamine Explosure Alters Immune Function in Normal and Retrovirus-infected Mice. *International Immunopharmacology*, June 2002, 2(7): 951–62.

Zernike, K. With Scenes of Blood and Pain, Ads Battle Methamphetamine in Montana. *New York Times*, February 26, 2006. http://www.nytimes.com/2006/02/06/natinal/26meth/hmtl?_r=1&oref=login.

Zickler, Patrick. Brain Activity Patterns Signal Risk of Relapse to Methamphetamine. *NIDA Notes*. 2006, 20(5): 1–6.

Zweben, J. F.; Cohen, J. B.; Christian, D.; Galloway, G. P.; Salinardi, M, Parent, D.; Iguchi, M; and Methamphetamine Treatment Project. Psychiatric Symptoms in Methamphetamine Users. *American Journal of Addiction*, March–April 2005, 13(2): 181–90.

ACKNOWLEDGMENTS

THANK YOU, JW, for being a wise role model who quietly and gently encouraged me throughout my life. I am grateful to the many individuals who were brave and generous enough to share their valuable experiences and wisdom, which I have tried in this book to share with others. Thank you to my many colleagues and mentors, including Petros Levounis and Marc Galanter, who helped me to persevere and galvanized me to start this project, which I personally felt was so vital. I give my deep appreciation to family and friends who have been their patience, encouragement, and support. And, of course, thank you, RK and AT for showing me that through that special combination—the courage to push forward together with the acceptance of the limitations life gives us—we can accomplish anything, including controlling addiction and finding happiness in life.

INDEX

destigmatize, 301
detoxing, 102–10, 301
  See also withdrawal
Dexedrine, 28, 105
diazepam, 103
digestive system, 36
diphenhydramine, 106
discussing addiction, 134–37, 279–84
doctors, 108–10
dopamine
  and addiction, 157, 160, 164
  antagonists, 159
  defined, 28, 35, 301
  effects of crystal meth, 30–32, 35, 51, 104
  schizophrenia, 39
  transporters, 31, 301
dope-sick, 301
dry mouth, 34
DSM-IV (*The Diagnostic and Statistical Manual of Mental Disorders*), 45, 47, 301
  attention-deficit/hyperactivity disorder criteria, 212–14
  depression criteria, 204–5
  dysthymia criteria, 206
  social phobia, 189
dual diagnosis, 162–65
dysthymia, 205–7, 302
  See also depression

E

Ecstasy, 18, 198, 302, 304
ego, 265
electrolytes, 302
emergency room visits, 26
employment, 208–10
ephedra, 30
ephedrine, 30
ERP (exposure with response prevention), 196–97
Eskalith, 165
ether, 40
euphoric recall, 79, 81
expectations, 171–87

F

family members, 278–90
Federal Controlled Substance Act of 1970, 16
fertilizer, 40
FIV (feline immunodeficiency virus), 271–72, 274
flumazenil, 161
Focalin, 30, 105
free radicals, 31, 302
Freud, Sigmund, 200
friends, 230–46
  addicted, 278–90
frontal cortex, 302

G

GABA (gamma-aminobutyric acid), 157
GABA receptors, 104, 161
gabapentin, 158
Gabitril, 159
Galanter, Marc, xi–xiii
gay men
  drug use, 7, 11, 17–22, 65
  parental expectations, 174
  party scene, 231–32
  psychological considerations, 53
(GVG) gamma-vinyl GABA, 159
Geodon, 165
GHB (gamma-hydroxybutyrate), 105, 302
ginseng, 30
glossary, 297–311
glutamate, 51, 160, 302
Grant, I., 65
guarana, 30
gum chewing, 93

H

HAART (highly active anti-retroviral treatment), 275, 303
Haldol, 165
hallucinations, 39, 302
haloperidol, 165
Halsted, William, xii

harm-reduction, 88–89, 302–3
  resources, 295–96
heart, 35–36
helper T-cells, 272, 303
heroin, xii, 53
heterosexual men, 27, 65
high-risk situations, 118–21, 131
HIV, 27, 268–76
  and immune system, 101
  medications, 91, 161, 274–76
  transmission of, 6–7, 20, 248
homosexuality. *See* gay men
honeymoon period, 79
Humphries, 142
hydroxazine, 106
hyperactivity, 213
hypothalamus, 303

I

id, 265
immune system, 272–73, 303
impulsivity, 213
in vitro, 303
in vivo, 303
inattention, 213
ingredients of crystal methamphet-
    amine, 16, 40–42
  purity of, 42
injecting crystal, 20, 32, 92
inpatient programs, 149–55
inpatient rehabilitation, 303
insight, 303
insurance companies, 153
internet, 119–20
  recipes for crystal, 41
  resources, 291–96
  sex sites, 20
IOPs (intensive outpatient programs),
    145–46

J

JCAHO (Joint Commission on
    Accreditation of Healthcare
    Organizations), 151–52
jetlag, 50
"Just Say No", 73, 121, 146

K

Kemstro, 159
ketamine, 18, 303
Khantzian, Edward, 243
kidneys, 36
killer T-cells, 272, 304
kindling effect, 39
Klonopin, 103, 199
Kübler-Ross, Elisabeth, 267

L

Lamictal, 165
lamotrigine, 165
lead, 42
lifestyles, 118, 130
limbic system, 304
line, 304
lithium, 40, 165
Lithobid, 165
loneliness, 230–46
lorazepam, 103–4
loss of control, 48
lubricants, 94–95
Lunesta, 106
lymphocyte, 304
Lyrica, 104

M

ma huang, 30
major depression, 203–4, 207, 304
  See also depression
manufacture of crystal meth, 16, 40–42
  purity of, 42
MAOIs (monoamine oxidase inhibi-
    tors), 275
Maragos, William F., 274
marijuana receptors, 157
Marlatt, G. Alan, 67, 116
massage, 223–25
Matrix Model, 148–49, 304
McKellar, 142
MDMA (methylenedioxymethamphet-
    amine), 198, 304
medications, 156–62
  HIV, 274–76

social anxiety, 198–200
withdrawal, 103–10
meditation, 227–29
melatonon receptors, 106
mercury, 41
mesolimbic pathway, 32, 49, 304
Metadate, 30, 105
meth labs, 41
meth mouth, 34, 93, 95, 304
methamphetamine. *See* crystal methamphetamine
methanol, 40
methyl group, 28
methylene, 41
methylphenidate, 30, 105, 211
Mexico, 41, 42
military, 15–16
modafinil, 105–6, 159–61, 305
Moos, 142
Mormons, 7
morphine, xii
motorcycle gangs, 16
mu-opiod receptor, 305
muriatic acid, 40
muscles, 36–37
mushin, 305
mutations, 305

N

NA (Narcotics Anynymous), 143
naltrexone, 158, 305
National Survey of Substance Abuse
   Treatment Services, 151–52
natural remedies, 30, 96
needles, 92
negative emotions, 128–30
neocortex, 50, 305
nephrons, 36
Neurontin, 158
neurophysiologic, 305
neurotransmitter, 30, 305
NMDA (N-methyl-D-aspartic acid),
   157, 305
nonoxynol-9, 94, 305–6
norepinephrine, 28, 164, 306
Norvir, 274

nucleus accumbens, 32, 306
nutrition, 96

O

obesity, 66
olanzapine, 165
oral sex, 95
organizations, 291–96
osteoporosis, 34
overdose, 38–39
oxcarbazepine, 165

P

paranoia, 39, 306
parents, 174–76
Parkinson's disease, 38, 306
partners, 288–90
Patterson, T.L., 65
pemoline, 30, 105
PET (positron emission tomography)
   scans, 37–38, 125, 306
physical dependence, 53–54
physiological dependence, 47
PI (protease inhibitors), 161
placebo, 162, 306
PNP (party and play), 20, 306
precautions using crystal meth, 92
prefrontal cortex, 306
pregabalin, 104
pregnancy, 24–25
primitive brain, 49–50
the program, 307
Prometa, 161–62
protease inhibitor, 307
Provigil, 105–6, 159, 307
pseudoephedrine, 40, 42
psychiatric illnesses, 162–65
psychodynamic psychotherapy, 200–
   201, 307
psychological relief, 52
psychology, 306
psychosis, 39, 307
purity of crystal meth, 42